ANTIBIOTICS

ANTIBIOTICS

The Comprehensive Guide

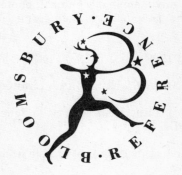

BLOOMSBURY

CONSULTANTS AND CONTRIBUTORS

Members of the Pharmocology Group, King's College London:
Dr Ian K. M. Morton BSc, PhD (Series Consultant)
Dr John Halliday BSc, PhD (Consultant)
Dr Judith M. Hall BSc, PhD (Technical Editor)
Alyson Fox BSc

First published 1990

Copyright © 1990 by Clark Robinson Limited

Bloomsbury Publishing Limited, 2 Soho Square, London W1V 5DE

The CIP record for this book is available from the British Library.

ISBN 0 7475 0623 X

Designed by Malcolm Smythe
Typeset by Action Typesetting Limited, Gloucester
Printed in Great Britain by
Richard Clay Ltd, Bungay, Suffolk

PREFACE

This dictionary is a comprehensive guide to the range of
antibiotics that are available in the United Kingdom
today. It also includes other drugs that are used to treat
infection (such as antiviral agents and antiparasitic drugs)
and vaccines. It is not intended to be a guide to the
prescription or administration of drugs; a qualified
practitioner should always be consulted before any
medicine is taken.

How to use this book
The book begins with an introduction to antibiotics and
allied drugs in general. Consulting it will enable the
reader to understand the factors that determine choices of
antibiotic therapy. This is followed by the A to Z. The
articles in the A to Z describe the antibiotics and other
drugs listed under their generic and proprietary names.
There are also articles describing the major drug types
(indicated by *).

The A to Z is cross-referenced so that further
information may be found quickly. Cross-references are
indicated by SMALL CAPITALS. Many of the articles list
warnings (indicated by ✚) about the use of a particular
drug, and a description the possible side-effects (indicated
by ▲).

INTRODUCTION

This book provides an essential quick reference for anyone
with an interest in the powerful drugs that are available
to treat or prevent infections and infectious diseases.
Naturally, different people are interested in different
things, depending on their circumstances. Parents
probably want to know about the vaccinations and
antibiotics that might be given to their children. People
travelling to tropical countries want to find out about any
injections or drugs they should take to guard against
serious and potentially deadly tropical diseases, such as
malaria. Someone with a relative who has had major
surgery may be anxious about the drugs used to treat a
post-operative infection which is hindering recovery. It is
to such varying groups of people that this book is
addressed.

The health of the society we now live in owes an
enormous amount to the effectiveness of the vaccination
programmes that have been carried out as a matter of
routine since the 1950s and earlier. The control of
appalling diseases which used to kill thousands every
year, such as diphtheria, tuberculosis and polio, and the
banishment of smallpox, are all triumphs of the
vaccination technique.

The development of a wide range of powerful antibiotics
means that many previously life-threatening conditions
can now successfully be treated. Many advances in
medical science have depended to a considerable degree on

the use of antibiotics, for example, organ transplants would be much more hazardous - perhaps even impossible - without the protection antibiotics give to the patient.

Despite our considerable progress, however, the battle against infection and infectious disease is by no means over. There are persistent outbreaks of such diseases as meningitis, Legionnaires' disease, listeriosis and salmonellosis, and frequent reports of hospital wards being closed because of drug-resistant infections. The ever-growing number of AIDS cases is an even more potent reminder that some inhabitants of the microbial kingdom are far from vanquished.

Generic and proprietary drugs

A doctor who prescribes a certain drug writes a prescription with the name of the medicine, its form (such as capsules or a cream), the dosage, the frequency of dosing and the duration of the treatment.

The name written on the prescription could be that of the drug itself; this is known as the "generic" or "chemical-" name. Alternatively, it could be the brand or trade name of a preparation of the drug; this is known as a "proprietary" name. Confusingly, the proprietary name of a preparation may bear no relation to the generic name of the drug it contains, because it is simply the name registered by the company marketing the preparation. A proprietary preparation of this type may be protected by patent. Doctors in the National Health Service are often encouraged to prescribe the generic forms of drugs, if they are available, because they are usually cheaper.

The generic name of the active drug in a proprietary medicine is not always shown on the container. Readers will find this book particularly useful because it provides an easy way of finding out what a prescribed medicine actually contains. If a generic drug has been prescribed, all readers have to do is look up the entry under that name in the dictionary, where they will find a description of the drug's uses, its contraindications, its possible side-effects, and warnings about its use. If the drug is a member of a larger family of drugs, there will also be a further entry under the family name, which provides more general information about that group of drugs.

If a proprietary medicine has been prescribed, the first step is to look up the entry under its proprietary name. This will give information about the manufacturer, the uses of the medicine, the forms in which the medicine is available and the generic name of the active drug or drugs the proprietary medicine contains. Looking up the generic name then gives access to further information, including possible side-effects.

What is an infection?

An infection occurs when the body's tissues or cells are invaded and damaged by foreign organisms. Such disease-causing organisms are called "pathogens", and most are members of the microbial kingdom. They are so tiny they can be seen only with the help of a microscope, and are often referred to as micro-organisms. Micro-organisms that cause infection include: viruses (the smallest and simplest); bacteria; chlamydia, rickettsiae, mycoplasma (all similar to bacteria); protozoa (single-celled animals) and fungi. Infection may also be caused by larger organisms such as parasitic worms (helminths), scabies mites and lice.

Infections cause disease by various mechanisms. First, the invading organisms may compete with the body's cells for nutrients. Second, they often provoke an intense reaction from the body's own defence mechanisms (the immune system), which results in the destruction of some of the body's cells as well as those of the invading organism. Third, the breakdown products of damaged micro-organisms often have toxic effects on the human host, resulting in fevers, the lowering of blood pressure and other dangerous adverse effects. Fourth, the micro-organisms may release poisonous substances (toxins) as they grow; tetanus is an example of a potentially lethal condition caused by bacteria that release a toxin from the site of an infected wound.

The major types of agents used to fight infections

Most agents in the dictionary can be classified into one of four types.

Antiseptics and **disinfectants** kill or slow the growth of micro-organisms on the surface of the body or in places such as kitchens and lavatories, where harmful micro-organisms can flourish. They are, however, toxic to human cells as well, and would cause serious tissue damage if injected or taken orally.

Vaccines are given before an infection occurs to stimulate the body's immune system into being able to recognize and inactivate either the infectious organism or any toxin it produces.

Antitoxins and **immunoglobulins** are preparations of antibodies that can neutralize toxins released by micro-organisms, or in the case of some immunoglobulins, the micro-organism itself. If injected, these can provide a degree of instant protection to a susceptible patient.

Selectively toxic drugs inhibit or kill an invading organism while causing little or no damage to the human host. These drugs are usually described by the prefix "anti-" followed by a word describing the type of organism concerned; for example, antifungals are used to treat fungal infections. Antibiotics are the largest group of drugs in this category.

What is an antibiotic?
The original, scientifically exact definition of an antibiotic is a chemical substance that is released by a micro-organism and that inhibits the growth of micro-organisms of a different species. However, the term has been popularized to mean any drug that is used to treat infections caused by bacteria and similar organisms, such as rickettsiae, chlamydia and mycoplasma. It is this popular usage that has been adopted throughout this book. This allows to us to group drugs of similar activity together, whether they are natural products or purely synthetic ones. It also means there will be no coverage of those natural products which, although antibiotic in the strict sense, are also highly toxic to human cells. (It is interesting to note that some drugs of this type are used as anticancer agents.)

How do antibiotics work?

Antibiotics and similar drugs act by exploiting differences between the structure or function of the invading micro-organism and that of the cells of the human host. This selective toxicity to an invading organism is characteristic of all successful antibiotics and similar drugs. For example, antibiotics of the penicillin family kill sensitive bacteria by inhibiting the formation of the bacterial cell wall, a structure that is essential to bacteria but is not present in human cells. Thus penicillin-type antibiotics have a potent effect on bacteria and relatively little toxicity to human cells.

Other common ways antibiotics work are by disrupting the processes of protein synthesis or disturbing the replication of the genetic material in the invading organism. These biological processes differ between human cells and pathogenic micro-organisms, and so the antibiotic can affect the micro-organism but not the patient. Examples are tetracyclines, aminoglycosides and erythromycin, which disrupt bacterial protein synthesis, and rifampicin, the quinolones and metronidazole, which inhibit gene function in bacteria.

Taking of antibiotics

To be effective, antibiotics must get to the site of the infection and be present in sufficient amounts for long enough to kill the micro-organisms or at least to weaken them enough for the patient's defences to complete the job. The blood and tissue fluid surrounding cells is the most efficient route to get an antibiotic to infected tissue. Therefore what is known as "systemic administration" is usually the best way of administering the drug. Systemic administration means giving the drug by mouth or by injection so that it is absorbed and distributed throughout the body by the blood and tissue fluids.

The most convenient way to give antibiotics is by mouth, but some antibiotics are not well absorbed by this means. For these drugs, injections must be used. Injections can also have the advantage of giving larger doses with a more rapid effect. Sometimes, a special poorly soluble preparation of an antibiotic is injected into the muscle so that it is gradually released over a number of days; this is known as a depot injection.

With very young children, who cannot swallow tablets or capsules, there may be difficulties in getting them to accept some antibiotic syrups because they dislike the taste. In such a situation a different preparation (perhaps sweetened or flavoured) or even an alternative antibiotic with an acceptable taste may be tried. Some antibiotics are available in a concentrated liquid form that can be administered by a small plastic dropper tube straight into the mouth, avoiding some of the difficulties of giving an infant a large volume from a spoon.

In order to maintain a sufficient concentration of antibiotic in the blood it is important to balance the rate of breakdown or excretion of the drug with the rate of administration. Many antibiotics, such as the penicillins, are very rapidly excreted by the kidneys, and to make up for this doses have to be given several times during the day. Missing a dose or two can allow the micro-organisms to flourish again, delaying an eventual cure. For a similar reason, it is very important to complete a course of treatment; even if the infection seems much improved it may flourish again if the patient stops taking the antibiotic too soon.

The presence of food in the stomach can inhibit the absorption of some antibiotics that have been taken by mouth. It is therefore recommended that these drugs are taken on an empty stomach, perhaps half an hour before a meal. Ampicillin, some preparations of erythromycin and some tetracyclines are examples of such antibiotics. With many antibiotics it is of little consequence whether the preparation is taken before, during or after meals. However, levels of the antibiotic in the blood will usually reach a higher peak if the drug is taken on an empty stomach. Taking some antibiotics on a full stomach, on the other hand, may lessen any gastric irritation they might cause.

Fairly equal spacing of doses during the day and taking the preparation on an empty stomach is usually the best advice for maintaining the most effective level of the drug in the blood to fight an infection.

There is a widely held belief that antibiotics and alcohol do not "mix". In fact, there are relatively few antibiotics that cause real problems if alcohol is also consumed. Ones that do cause problems are cephamandole, latamoxef, metronidazole, nimorazole and tinidazole, which all inhibit the metabolism of alcohol. This leads to the accumulation in the body of a toxic substance called acetaldehyde, which causes symptoms of flushing, headache, palpitations, nausea and vomiting.

Except when taking one of the five antibiotics mentioned, a modest intake of alcohol is unlikely to cause trouble. Alcohol does, however, put a strain on the liver and perhaps depresses some immune mechanisms, neither of which is helpful when fighting off an infection.

Which organism is responsible for an infection?

Before treatment of an infection can be started, an assessment of which micro-organism is causing the infection must be made. The initial assessment depends largely on the diagnostic skills of the doctor. In some cases the symptoms and history of the illness make diagnosis fairly easy, but often there are a number of possible micro-organisms that could be the culprit. For example, urinary tract infections, pneumonia and meningitis can each be caused by a number of micro-organisms, many of which may be attacked by different antibiotics. The exact micro-organism can be confirmed by sending a specimen of infected material to a bacteriology laboratory. This is an expensive and time-consuming process, however, and not justified when treating uncomplicated minor infections. But if an infection persists for longer than expected despite treatment, or if the infection is serious, laboratory investigation is usually to be recommended.

Gram staining

There is an important means of identifying and classifying bacteria that should be mentioned, which is the laboratory technique called gram staining. Most bacteria can be readily classified by this staining procedure as either gram-positive or gram-negative, although there are exceptions. Gram-positive bacteria stain blue/purple and gram-negative bacteria stain pink/red. The difference in staining represents differences in the properties of the cell wall of these two types of bacteria. There is frequently a correlation between the gram-staining characteristic of a bacterium and its sensitivity to various families of antibiotics. By way of example, the early penicillins are active primarily against gram-positive organisms, whereas aminoglycosides are most useful in the treatment of gram-negative infections.

When should an antibiotic be used?
In many cases antibiotic therapy is clearly appropriate and its benefits can easily be seen. But often the case for using antibiotics is far from straightforward, particularly when treating colds, sore throats and coughs. Most of these infections are caused by viruses, and are dealt with by the body's immune system within a week or two. Antibiotics do not have any effect upon the viruses responsible. However, antibiotics are beneficial if the illness is caused by a bacterial infection (for example, bacterial tonsillitis) or if there is a secondary bacterial infection (such as an infection of the ear following a viral common cold infection).

Which drug should be prescribed?
If a viral infection is diagnosed, the options available for drug treatment are somewhat restricted. Antiviral agents are few in number and most of them have only a limited effect or are rather toxic.

If micro-organisms other than viruses, such as bacteria or protozoa, are diagnosed, then the prospects of successful treatment by drugs are much more hopeful. Long experience, both in the laboratory and in the clinic, has shown that different micro-organisms show characteristic patterns of sensitivity to particular drugs. For example, the type of streptococcus that is the commonest cause of bacterial throat infections is, in a pure culture, always sensitive to the original penicillin, penicillin G. The situation is often more complicated, but nevertheless there are recognized first-choice drugs and often satisfactory alternatives for treating the great majority of non-viral infections.

If the infecting organism is definitely identified by laboratory investigation, so much the better. Such investigations can also test an organism's sensitivity to antibiotics, and allow a well-informed choice of drug. A speedy laboratory test of antibiotic sensitivity can be life-saving for a patient with a serious and rapidly developing infection.

How long should treatment last?

An infection is said to have been cured if there is no reappearance of the infection when the antibiotic therapy finishes. Thus an absence of relapse is the ultimate measure of the success of a treatment.

The duration of a treatment is determined by many considerations. Usually the nature of the infection and the organism responsible are the most important factors. For example, antibiotic treatment for tuberculosis takes between six and nine months, whereas a typical middle-ear infection may require only three days of treatment. Another important factor is the efficiency of a patient's own immune system. A healthy person's immune system rapidly overcomes micro-organisms that have been weakened by drug treatment, but patients with deficient immune responses require more potent and prolonged antibiotic therapy. The problem is that if too short a course is prescribed, some patients may relapse, whereas too long a course increases the risk of drug-resistant organisms developing (as explained below).

Might frequent use of antibiotics be a bad thing?

It is often said that taking antibiotics hinders the development of one's own immunity and that it is better to fight off infections without recourse to drugs. However, there is no strong scientific case to support this belief, and it should never deter anyone from justifiable treatment.

Serious or chronic infections can develop if a condition is not treated, and these can be much more of a problem than any, quite probably imagined, harm caused by antibiotics.

The idea that antibiotics can depress natural immunity probably arose from a confusion between this and two thoroughly substantiated facts. First, if an infection is viral, antibiotics will not help in its treatment. Second, long-term treatment with the same antibiotic greatly increases the chance of drug-resistant organisms emerging, which means that the antibiotic will cease to be effective.

Antibiotic resistance
Resistance develops when a strain of micro-organisms is frequently exposed to a particular antibiotic. In the presence of the antibiotic the resistant forms of the micro-organism survive and multiply, and so gradually become the dominant population. Only in the absence of the antibiotics concerned will these resistant forms decline again in numbers.

Frequently, "resistance factors" (carried by small rings of genetic material called plasmids) are transferred from one micro-organism to another, and can confer immediate resistance to the second organism. Sometimes resistance to several antibiotics can be transferred at once.

One mechanism of resistance involves the production by the bacterium of enzymes that inactivate the antibiotic by changing its chemical structure. Another mechanism is for the micro-organism to pump the antibiotic out if its cell as soon as it enters, preventing the concentration of the antibiotic in the cell from reaching an effective level. Yet another mechanism is for the micro-organism to alter the structure of the part of its cell that the antibiotic attacks, so that the antibiotic is no longer effective.

The phenomenon of resistance is an important one and has seriously limited the usefulness of many previously effective antibiotics. The problem is particularly severe in hospitals where saturation of the environment with antibiotics encourages resistant strains to emerge and multiply.

The best defences are to use antibiotics sparingly, to use narrow-spectrum antibiotics (which affect only a limited number of micro-organisms) whenever possible, and to change antibiotics before resistant strains have a chance to emerge.

Why might antibiotic treatment fail?

There are several reasons for the failure of antibiotic treatment. Sometimes it is because a virus and not a bacterium is the infecting organism, or an unusual micro-organism is responsible for the infection and is not affected by the chosen antibiotic. But very often it is because the infection is caused by a resistant strain of a normally sensitive bacterium, as described above.

A rather different problem is the presence of a foreign body in a wound, or the insertion of a surgical implant, both of which can greatly hinder the eradication of infection at the site. A collection of pus at the site of an abscess can also greatly interfere with the access of the antibiotic to the infected tissue, and thus reduce the antibiotic's efficacy. Occasionally, an unexplained failure of treatment may be caused by an unsuspected deficiency in the patient's immune system.

Adverse reactions to antibiotics and similar drugs

There are three main types of adverse reactions. First, there are direct toxic effects. For example, prolonged treatment with high doses of an aminoglycoside antibiotic (such as streptomycin) can cause damage to the auditory nerves and so to hearing.

The second type of reaction is a hypersensitivity (allergic reaction) to the drug. This is the commonest type of adverse reaction to penicillins. Such reactions are usually slight, but some patients have severe reactions, known as anaphylactic shock, which make the use of the drug in question very dangerous. This is why doctors must be very careful to find out if the patient has ever suffered a reaction to a drug in the past before prescribing. If such reactions have occurred, an alternative drug of a different chemical family must be prescribed.

The third type of reaction is peculiar to antibiotics. It happens because antibiotics may also kill off the harmless bacteria that normally live in the intestine and vagina, as well as the harmful bacteria they are intended to kill. The alteration in the normal range of bacteria found in these regions is often of little consequence, causing only the mild diarrhoea or vaginal thrush that often accompanies antibiotic treatment. But sometimes it allows an infection, known as a "superinfection", by other dangerous organisms that are not attacked by the antibiotic in use (a good example of this is the colitis that occasionally follows treatment with clindamycin). If this happens, another antibiotic may be needed to deal with an infection more serious than the original one.

In this dictionary, adverse reactions are listed as side-effects in the entry for each generic drug.

Contraindications
Sometimes there are specific reasons for not prescribing a particular drug, or for exercising caution if doing so. Such reasons are known as "contraindications" and are listed as warnings in the dictionary. For example, tetracycline antibiotics are contraindicated in children because they cause discoloration of growing teeth. There are also a number of drugs that should not be given to pregnant women. In some cases this is because there is an established risk of damaging the unborn baby, but more often it is simply because research with animals or theoretical considerations make it impossible to exclude a risk that damage might occur. Obviously in such circumstances it is unjustifiable to prescribe certain drugs if safe alternatives are available. In other cases there is merely insufficient positive evidence of the drug's safety and it is therefore suggested the drug should not be used in pregnancy because the risk is not known. In general antibiotics are relatively free of known adverse effects in pregnancy, but certain of the antifungal agents and antiviral agents do present a risk and should be avoided.

Another high-risk situation occurs when treating a patient who has poor kidney function with a drug that is normally excreted by the kidney and is known to be toxic at high dosage. A standard dosage for such a patient results in an accumulation of the drug to toxic levels because the kidneys are not extracting it at the normal rate. A similar situation can arise in treating a patient with liver damage if the drug is normally broken down or excreted by the liver.

Perhaps the commonest contraindication to an antibiotic is the patient having a history of hypersensitivity reactions to the drug or a drug in the same chemical class, as discussed above.

The future

Since the development of synthetic antibacterial compounds (the sulphonamides in the 1930s and the introduction of penicillin G into clinical practice in 1941) a host of new antibiotics have arrived on the scene. Most of these, however, have been modifications of existing antibiotics and, effective though many of these are, few represent radical new approaches. Now, however, the growth of techniques of molecular biology promises new insights into the biochemical processes of micro-organisms and their interactions with human cells. These insights will surely lead to the design of more effective and less toxic antibiotics and antiviral agents. New antibiotic-resistant strains of bacteria and protozoa are constantly emerging, however, and careful husbandry of our existing antibiotic resources is still needed to keep these organisms in check. There is much reason for optimism, and these are no less exciting times than those of the early pioneers in the field of antibiotics.

Dr John Halliday
Lecturer in Pharmacology
King's College London

Achromycin (*Lederle*) is a proprietary form of the broad-spectrum ANTIBIOTIC tetracycline hydrochloride, available only on prescription. Used to treat many types of microbial infections both systemically and on the skin and in the ears and eyes (notably to treat trachoma), Achromycin is produced in many forms: as tablets (in two types), as a syrup, as an ointment (in two strengths), as an ophthalmic oil suspension (for use as drops), and powdered in vials for reconstitution and injection. Some forms are not recommended for children or pregnant women.

▲/✚ side-effects/warning: *see* TETRACYCLINE.

Achromycin V (*Lederle*) is a form of the proprietary tetracycline ANTIBIOTIC Achromycin that also contains a buffer — a substance that does not change its acid-alkali balance (pH) if it is diluted. Produced in the form of capsules and as a syrup, it is not recommended for children or pregnant women.

▲/✚ side-effects/warning: *see* TETRACYCLINE.

Aci-Jel (*Ortho-Cilag*) is a proprietary, non-prescription, ANTISEPTIC preparation used to treat non-specific vaginal infections and restore acidity to the vagina. Produced in the form of a jelly (accompanied by a special applicator), Aci-Jel's active constituent is acetic acid, which has an antibacterial activity.

▲ side-effects: there may be local irritation and/or inflammation.

acrosoxacin is an ANTIBIOTIC agent of the quinolone family used to treat the sexually-transmitted disease gonorrhoea in patients who are allergic to penicillin, or whose strain of gonorrhoea is resistant to penicillin-type antibiotics. Administration is oral in the form of capsules. It is not recommended for children.

▲ side-effects: there may be dizziness, drowsiness and headache such as to interrupt concentration or intricacy of movement or thought; there may also be gastrointestinal disturbances.

✚ warning: acrosoxacin should be administered with caution to epileptics, or patients who have impaired kidney or liver function, or who are pregnant or breast feeding.
Related article: ERADACIN.

AC vax (*SK&F*) is a VACCINE designed to give protection against the organism meningococcus, which can cause serious infection including meningitis. It may be indicated for travellers intending to go to parts of the world where the risk of meningococcal infection is much higher than in the United Kingdom, e.g. parts of Africa. It may be given to adults and children over two months.

acyclovir is an ANTIVIRAL agent used specifically to treat infection by herpes viruses (such as shingles, chickenpox, cold sores including genital sores, and herpes infections of the eye). It works by inhibiting the action of two virally coded enzymes in cells used by the virus to replicate itself. To be effective, however, treatment of an infection must begin early. It may be valuable in immunocompromised patients. The drug may also be used prophylactically to prevent individuals at risk from contracting a herpes disease. Administration is oral, topical or by infusion.
▲ side-effects: applied topically, there may be a temporary burning or stinging sensation; some patients experience a localized drying of the skin. Taken orally, acyclovir may give rise to gastrointestinal disturbance and various blood cell deficiencies; there may also be fatigue and a rash.
✚ warning: acyclovir should be administered with caution to patients who are pregnant or who have impaired kidney function. To be effective, treatment of an infection must begin as early as possible. Adequate fluid intake must be maintained.
Related article: ZOVIRAX.

adsorbed diphtheria and tetanus vaccine is diphtheria

and tetanus VACCINE adsorbed on to a mineral carrier.
see DIPHTHERIA AND TETANUS VACCINE.

adsorbed diphtheria, tetanus and pertussis vaccine is
diphtheria, pertussis (whooping cough) and tetanus (DPT)
VACCINE adsorbed on to a mineral carrier.
see DIPHTHERIA, PERTUSSIS AND TETANUS (DPT) VACCINE.

adsorbed tetanus vaccine is tetanus VACCINE adsorbed on
to a mineral carrier.
see TETANUS VACCINE.

Aerosporin (*Calmic*) is a proprietary form of the
ANTIBIOTIC drug polymyxin B sulphate, available only on
prescription, which is active against gram-negative
bacteria. It is produced in the form of powder for
reconstitution as a medium for injections.
▲/✚ side-effects/warning: *see* POLYMYXIN B SULPHATE.

Albucid (*Nicholas*) is a proprietary ANTIBIOTIC of the
SULPHONAMIDE family, available only on prescription, used
to treat eye infections. Produced in the form of eye-drops
and (under the trade name Albucid Ointment) as an
ointment (in either a water-miscible base or an oily base),
Albucid's active constituent is the sulphonamide
sulphacetamide sodium.
▲/✚ side-effects/warning: *see* SULPHACETAMIDE.

Alcobon (*Roche*) is a proprietary ANTIFUNGAL drug
available only on prescription, used to treat systemic
infections by yeasts (such as candidiasis, or thrush).
Produced for hospital use only in the form of tablets
and in infusion flasks, Alcobon is a preparation of
flucytosine.
▲/✚ side-effects/warning: *see* FLUCYTOSINE.

alcohol is the name of a class of compounds derived from
hydrocarbons. For medical purposes, a strong solution of
ethyl alcohol can be used as an ANTISEPTIC (particularly to
prepare skin before injection) or as a preservative.

Alcopar (*Wellcome*) is a proprietary non-prescription ANTHELMINTIC drug, used to treat infections by roundworms, specifically by hookworms. Produced in the form of granules in sachets for solution in water, Alcopar is a preparation of bephenium hydroxynaphthoate.
▲ side-effects: *see* BEPHENIUM.

Almevax (*Wellcome*) is a proprietary VACCINE against German measles (rubella) in the form of a solution containing live but attenuated viruses of the Wistar RA27/3 strain. Available only on prescription, and administered in the form of injection, it is intended specifically for the immunization of non-pregnant women.

Almodan (*Berk*) is a proprietary ANTIBIOTIC available only on prescription, used to treat systemic bacterial infections of the upper respiratory tract, of the ear, of the sinuses and of the urogenital tracts; it is sometimes used to treat typhoid fever. Produced in the form of capsules, as a syrup for dilution and as a powder for reconstitution as a medium for injection, Almodan is a preparation of the broad-spectrum penicillin amoxycillin.
▲/✚ side-effects/warning: *see* AMOXYCILLIN.

aluminium acetate is an astringent DISINFECTANT, used primarily to clean sites of infection and inflammation, particularly in the case of weeping or suppurating wounds or sores, eczema, and infections of the outer ear. Administration is in the form of a lotion (containing aluminium acetate in dilute solution) or as drops.

amantadine hydrochloride is an ANTIVIRAL agent used to prevent infection with the influenza A2 virus (but not other types of influenza virus) and in the treatment of shingles. Administration is oral in the form of capsules or as a dilute syrup.
▲ side-effects: there is commonly restlessness and inability to concentrate; there may also be dizziness and insomnia, gastrointestinal disturbances, swelling resulting from fluid retention in the tissues, and skin

discoloration. A regular blood count is advisable.

✚ warning: amantadine should not be administered to patients who suffer from gastric ulcers or from epilepsy. It should be administered with caution to patients who suffer from heart, liver or kidney disease, psychosis, or long-term eczema; who are pregnant or lactating; who are in a state of confusion; or who are elderly. Withdrawal of treatment must be gradual.

Ambaxin (*Upjohn*) is a proprietary ANTIBIOTIC, available only on prescription, used to treat systemic bacterial infections and infections of the upper respiratory tract, the ear, nose and throat, and the urogenital tracts. Produced in the form of tablets, Ambaxin is a preparation of the broad-spectrum penicillin bacampicillin.

▲/✚ side-effects/warning: *see* BACAMPICILLIN.

Amfipen (*Brocades*) is a proprietary ANTIBIOTIC, available only on prescription, used to treat systemic bacterial infections and infections of the upper respiratory tract, the ear, nose and throat, and the urogenital tracts. Produced in the form of capsules (in two strengths), as a powder for reconstitution, as a syrup (in two strengths, under the trade name Amfipen Syrup), and in vials for injection (in two strengths, under the name Amfipen Injection), Amfipen is a preparation of the broad-spectrum penicillin ampicillin.

▲/✚ side-effects/warning: *see* AMPICILLIN.

amikacin is an ANTIBIOTIC drug (of the aminoglycoside family), used to treat several serious bacterial infections, particularly those due to gram-negative organisms that prove to be resistant to the more generally-used aminoglycosides GENTAMICIN and TOBRAMYCIN. Administration is by intramuscular or intravenous injection or infusion.

▲ side-effects: extended and/or high dosage may cause irreversible deafness; temporary kidney malfunction may occur.

✚ warning: amikacin should not be administered to

patients who are pregnant (because the drug can cross the placenta), and should be administered with caution to patients with impaired function of the kidney. Careful monitoring for toxicity is advisable during treatment.

Amikin (*Bristol-Myers*) is a proprietary preparation of the aminoglycoside ANTIBIOTIC amikacin, available only on prescription, used to treat several serious bacterial infections, particularly those that prove to be resistant to the more generally used aminoglycoside GENTAMICIN. Amikin is produced in vials for injection or infusion (as amikacin sulphate) in two strengths.
▲/✚ side-effects/warning: *see* AMIKACIN.

*amoebicidal drugs treat infection by the microscopic protozoan organisms known as amoebae, which cause such disorders as amoebic dysentery and hepatic amoebiasis. Best known and most used is metronidazole, both for acute intestinal forms of infection (amoebic dysentery) and amoebic abscesses of the liver. An alternative amoebicidal drug for this treatment is tinidazole. In cases in which ameobic cysts are being passed on defecation but there are no further symptoms in the patient, the drug of choice is diloxanide furoate.
▲/✚ side-effects/warning: *see* DILOXANIDE FUROATE; METRONIDAZOLE; TINIDAZOLE.
Related articles: AVLOCLOR; FLAGYL; FLAGYL S; FURAMIDE; METROLYL; NIDAZOL; ZADSTAT.

Amoxil (*Bencard*) is a proprietary ANTIBIOTIC, available only on prescription, used to treat systemic bacterial infections and infections of the upper respiratory tract, of the ear, nose and throat, and of the urogenital tracts; it is sometimes used also to treat typhoid fever. Produced in the form of capsules (in two strengths), as sugar-free soluble (dispersible) tablets, as a syrup for dilution (in two strengths; the potency of the syrup once diluted is retained for 14 days), as a suspension for children, in the form of powder in sachets, as a sugar-free powder in sachets, and as a powder in vials for reconstitution as a medium for injection, Amoxil is a preparation of the broad-spectrum PENICILLIN amoxycillin.

▲/✚ side-effects/warning: *see* AMOXYCILLIN.

amoxycillin is a broad-spectrum penicillin-type ANTIBIOTIC, closely related to AMPICILLIN. Readily absorbed orally, it is used to treat many infections, especially infections of the urogenital tracts, the upper respiratory tract, or the middle ear. It is also sometimes used to treat typhoid fever or to prevent infection following dental surgery. Administration is oral in the form of capsules or liquids, or by injection.

▲ side-effects: there may be sensitivity reactions such as rashes, high temperature and joint pain. Allergic patients may suffer anaphylactic shock. The most common side-effect, however, is diarrhoea.

✚ warning: amoxycillin should not be administered to patients who are known to be allergic to penicillin-type antibiotics; it should be administered with caution to those with impaired kidney function.
Related articles: AMOXIDIN; AMOXIL; AUGMENTIN.

amphotericin is a broad-spectrum ANTIFUNGAL agent used particularly to treat infection by fungal organisms. It can be given by infusion, and is extremely important in the treatment of systemic fungal infections and is active against almost all fungi and yeasts. However, it is a toxic drug and side-effects are common. Administration is oral in the form of tablets, lozenges or liquids, or by infusion.

▲ side-effects: treatment by infusion may cause nausea, vomiting, severe weight loss and ringing in the ears (tinnitus); some patients experience a marked reduction in blood potassium. Prolonged or high dosage may cause kidney damage.

✚ warning: amphotericin should not be administered to patients who are already undergoing drug treatment that may affect kidney function. During treatment by infusion, tests on kidney function are essential; the site of injection must be changed frequently.
Related articles: FUNGILIN; FUNGIZONE.

ampicillin is a broad-spectrum penicillin-type ANTIBIOTIC, orally absorbed — although absorption is reduced by the presence of food in the stomach or intestines — used to treat many infections and especially infections of the urogenital tracts, of the upper respiratory tract, or of the middle ear. Many bacteria have over the past two decades, however, become resistant to ampicillin. Administration is oral in the form of capsules or liquids, or by injection.

▲ side-effects: there may be sensitivity reactions such as rashes (invariably in patients suffering from glandular fever), high temperature and joint pain. Allergic patients may suffer anaphylactic shock. The most common side-effect, however, is diarrhoea.

✚ warning: ampicillin should not be administered to patients who are known to be allergic to penicillin-type antibiotics; in case anaphylactic shock ensues it should be administered with caution to those with impaired kidney function.

Related articles: AMPICLOX; AMPIFEN; BRITCIN; FLU-AMP; MAGNAPEN; PENBRITIN; VIDOPEN.

Ampiclox (*Beecham*) is a proprietary ANTIBIOTIC, available only on prescription, used to treat systemic bacterial infections and infections of the upper respiratory tract, of the ear, nose and throat, and of the urogenital tracts. Produced in vials for injection, Ampiclox is a compound preparation of the broad-spectrum penicillinase-sensitive AMPICILLIN and the penicillinase-resistant CLOXACILLIN. A smaller dose version (under the trade name Ampiclox Neonatal) is produced in the form of a sugar-free suspension and as a powder for reconstitution as a medium for injection, and is used to treat or prevent infections in newborn or premature babies.

▲/✚ side-effects/warning: *see* AMPICILLIN; CLOXACILLIN.

Anaflex (*Geistlich*) is a proprietary non-prescription ANTIMICROBIAL preparation used to treat fungal infections of the mouth and the throat, and also applied topically to treat many skin infections. Produced in the form of an aerosol spray, as a water-miscible cream, as a dusting-powder (with talc), as a paste, and in the form of lozenges (which are not recommended for children aged under 6 years); the aerosol, paste and powder should only be used externally. Anaflex is a preparation of the drug POLYNOXYLIN.

Antepar (*Wellcome*) is a proprietary non-prescription ANTHELMINTIC drug used to treat infestation by threadworms or roundworms. A laxative administered simultaneously is often expedient. Produced in the form of tablets and as an elixir for dilution (the potency of the elixir once diluted is retained for 14 days), Antepar is a preparation of piperazine hydrate.
▲/✚ side-effects/warning: *see* PIPERAZINE.

*anthelmintic drugs are used to treat infections by parasitic organisms of the helminth (worm) family. The threadworm, the roundworm and the tapeworm are the most common helminths responsible for infection in the UK. In warmer underdeveloped countries illness caused by helminths, e.g. hookworms (anaemia and debilitation), schistosomes (bilharzia) and filaria (elephantiasis and onchocerciasis) is a major health problem. Most worms infest the intestines; diagnosis often corresponds to evidence of their presence as shown in the faeces. Drugs can then be administered, and the worms are killed or anaesthetized and excreted in the normal way. Complications arise if the worms migrate within the body, in which case in order to make the environment in the body untenable for the worms, the treatment becomes severely unpleasant for the patient. In the case of threadworms, medication should be combined with hygienic measures (e.g. short finger nails) and the whole family should be treated. Among the most useful and best known anthelmintics are PIPERAZINE, MEBENDAZOLE, PRAZIQUANTEL, DIETHYLCARBAMAZINE and THIABENDAZOLE.

anthrax vaccine is generally required only by patients who are exposed to anthrax-infected hides and carcasses, or who handle imported bonemeal, fishmeal and feedstuffs. Available only on prescription, this inactivated bacterial vaccine consists of a suspension administered by injection in three doses over 9 weeks followed by another shot after 6 months; thereafter there may be an annual booster if necessary.

*antibacterial drugs have a selectively toxic action on bacteria. They can be used both topically, i.e. on the skin or the eye, to treat infections of superficial tissues or systemically, carried by the blood following absorbtion or injection, to the site of the infection. As bacteria are the largest and most diverse group of pathogenic micro-organisms, antibacterials form the major constituent group of ANTIBIOTICS.

*antibiotics are, strictly speaking, natural products secreted by micro-organisms into their environment where they inhibit the growth of competing micro-organisms of different species. But in common usage, and in this book, the term is applied to any drug – natural or synthetic – that has a selectively toxic action on bacteria or similar non-nucleated, single-celled micro-organisms (including chlamydia, rickettsia and mycoplasma); such drugs have no effect on viruses. Most synthetic antibiotics are modelled on natural substances. When administered by an appropriate route, such as orally, by injection or by infusion, antibiotics kill infective bacteria (bactericidal action) or inhibit their growth (bacteriostatic action). The selectively toxic action on invading bacteria exploits differences between bacteria and their human host cells. Major target sites are the bacterial cell wall located outside the cell membrane (human cells have only a cell membrane), and the bacterial ribosome (the protein-synthesizing organelle within its cell), which is different in bacteria and in human cells. Antibiotics of the PENICILLIN and CEPHALOSPORIN families (collectively known as beta-lactam antibiotics) attack the bacterial cell wall, whereas aminoglycoside and TETRACYCLINE antibiotics attack the bacterial ribosomes. Viruses, which lack both cell walls and ribosomes, are therefore resistant to these and other similar antibiotics.

Because there is such a diversity of disease-causing (pathogenic) bacteria, it is not surprising that specific infections are best treated using specific antibiotics, developed to combat them. But unfortunately, with the continuing widespread use of antibiotics, certain strains of common bacteria have developed resistance to antibiotics that were formerly effective against them. This is now a major problem. Another problem is the occurance of "superinfections", in which the use of a broad-spectrum antibiotic disturbs the normal, harmless bacterial population in the body as well as the pathogenic ones. In mild cases this may allow, for example, an existing but latent oral or vaginal thrush infection to become worse, or mild diarrhoea to develop. In rare cases the superinfection that develops is more serious than the disorder for which the antibiotic was administered.

*antifungal drugs are used to treat infections caused by fungal micro-organisms; they may be naturally or synthetically produced. Usually fungal infections are not a major problem in healthy, well-nourished individuals. However, superficial, localized infections such as thrush, caused by *Candida albicans*, and athlete's foot or ringworm, caused by fungi of the dermatophyte group, are common. Severe infections occur most frequently where the host's immunity is low, for example following immunosuppression for transplant surgery. Under such conditions fungi that are not normally pathogenic can exploit the situation and generate a life-threatening infection. Unfortunately the most potent antifungal drugs also tend to be highly toxic, and therefore severe systemic fungal infections remain a considerable danger. NYSTATIN and IMIDAZOLES such as CLOTRIMAZOLE are used for local treatment, with GRISEOFULVIN as an alternative. AMPHOTERICIN and FLUCYTOSINE are reserved for systemic fungal infections. The most common form of fungal infection in childhood is thrush. It usually occurs in the mouth and in the nappy area of infants. The treatment most often used involves topical nystatin or MICONAZOLE.

*antimalarial drugs are used to treat or prevent malaria. The disease is caused by infection of the red blood cells with a small organism called a protozoon (of the genus *Plasmodium*) which is carried by the Anopheles mosquito. Infection occurs as a result of the female mosquito's bite. The class of drug most frequently used to treat or prevent infection by the malaria protozoon are the quinidines, of which CHLOROQUINE is the standard. However, in some parts of the world, some forms of the protozoon that causes malaria are resistant to chloroquine; in such cases, the traditional remedy for malaria, QUININE, is used. Quinine may also be used in patients who cannot tolerate chloroquine. The prevention of malaria by drugs cannot be guaranteed. However, administration of chloroquine, PROGUANIL or PYRIMETHAMINE before, and for a period after, travelling to a tropical place, is thought to provide reasonable protection.

*antimicrobials are drugs used to treat infections caused by microbes. These include the major classes of pathogenic micro-organisms covered in this book — viruses, mycoplasma, rickettsia, chlamydia, protozoa, bacteria and fungi (but not helminths (worms)). Antimicrobial is therefore a wide term embracing ANTIBACTERIALS, ANTIBIOTICS, ANTIPROTOZOALS, ANTIVIRALS and ANTIFUNGALS. A drug that combines both the properties of an antibacterial and an antifungal could be more concisely termed an antimicrobial. However, in this text more specific terms are used where possible.

*antiprotozoal drugs are used to treat or prevent infections caused by micro-organisms called protozoa. Of these the most important, in terms of illness and death, are the protozoa of the genus *Plasmodium*, which cause malaria. Other major protozoal diseases found in tropical countries include trypanosomiasis, leishmaniasis and amoebic dysentery. Protozoal infections more familiar in this country include toxoplasmosis, trichomoniasis and giardiasis. A common form of pneumonia is caused in immunosuppressed patients (including those suffering from AIDS) by the protozoon *Pneumocytis carinii*.

see ANTIMALARIAL DRUGS

***antiseptics** are agents that destroy micro-organisms, or inhibit their activity to a level such that they are less or no longer harmful to health. Antiseptics may be applied to the skin, burns or wounds to prevent infections and to limit the spread of pathogenic micro-organisms. The term antiseptic is often used synonymously with DISINFECTANT.

***antiserum** is a general term used to describe certain preparations of blood serum rich in particular antibodies. Antiserums are used to provide (passive) immunity to diseases, or to provide some measure of treatment if the disease has already been contracted. The general term used to describe part of the disease-causing entity recognized by the immune system is "antigen". If an antigen is injected into an animal, the animal produces antibodies in response to the antigen. An antiserum is a sample of blood serum containing these antibodies. Most antiserums are prepared from blood of antigen-treated horses, and when the purified antiserums are used to immunize humans they often cause hypersensitivity reactions. For this reason use of such preparations is now very rare, and they have to a large extent been replaced by preparations of human antibodies.

***antitubercular** (or antituberculous) **drugs** are used in combination to treat tuberculosis. The initial phase of treatment usually employs three drugs (ordinarily ISONIAZID, RIFAMPICIN and PYRAZINAMIDE with STREPTOMYCIN or ETHAMBUTOL as possible alternatives) in order to tackle the disease as efficiently as possible, while reducing the risk of encountering bacterial resistance. If the first line of treatment is successful, after about 2 months treatment usually continues with only two of the initial three drugs (one of which is generally isoniazid).

If the first line of treatment was not successful, for example because the patient suffered intolerable side-effects or because the disease was resistant to drugs, then other drugs (e.g. CAPREOMYCIN and CYCLOSERINE) are used to treat the patient. The duration of treatment depends on the combination of drugs used.

***antiviral drugs** are relatively few in number and their effectiveness is often restricted to preventive or disease-limitation treatment. This is perhaps not surprising as viruses reproduce by taking over the biochemical machinery of the host cells and perverting it to their own needs. Therefore, it is extremely difficult to design a drug that can differentiate between attacking a vital viral mechanism and the host cell itself. However, some antiviral drugs can be lifesavers, especially in immunocompromised individuals. Infections due to the herpes viruses (e.g. cold sores, genital herpes and chicken pox) may be prevented or contained by early treatment with ACYCLOVIR. Serious cytomegaloviral infections may also be contained by treatment with ganciclovir. Severe respiratory infections in children are treated with ribavirin. As more of the molecular biology of the virus-host interactions becomes known, more selective antivirals are possible.

Apsin V.K. (*Approved Prescription Services*) is a proprietary ANTIBIOTIC, available only on prescription, used to treat bacterial infections of the skin and of the ear, nose and throat. It is similar to the original penicillin, penicillin G, though less active, but it does have the advantage of being orally absorbed. However, its absorbtion is too irregular for it to be recommended for treating severe infections. Produced in the form of tablets and as a syrup (in two strengths) for dilution (the potency of the syrup once dilute is retained for 7 days if stored at a temperature below 15 degrees centigrade), Apsin V.K. is a preparation of the PENICILLIN phenoxymethylpenicillin (penicillin V).

▲/✚ side-effects/warning: *see* PHENOXYMETHYLPENICILLIN.

Arilvax (*Wellcome*) is a proprietary form of VACCINE against yellow fever. It consists of a suspension containing live but weakened viruses, which are cultured in chick embryos. Available only on prescription, it is produced in vials with a diluent. It is not recommended for children under the age of 9 months.

✚ warning: see YELLOW FEVER VACCINE.

Arpimycin (*RP Drugs*) is a proprietary ANTIBIOTIC, available only on prescription, used both to treat many forms of infection (particularly pneumonia and legionnaires' disease) and to prevent others (particularly sinusitis, diphtheria and whooping cough); it is also used as an alternative to penicillin-type antibiotics in patients who are allergic or whose infections are resistant to penicillins. Produced in the form of a mixture (in three strengths) for dilution (the potency of the syrup once diluted is retained for 7 days), Arpimycin is a preparation of the macrolide antibiotic erythromycin.

▲/✚ side-effects/warning: *see* ERYTHROMYCIN.

Ascabiol (*May & Baker*) is a proprietary non-prescription preparation of BENZYL BENZOATE in suspension, used to treat infestation of the skin of the trunk and limbs by itch-mites (scabies) or sometimes to treat infestation by lice. A skin irritant, it is not suitable for use on the head, face and neck; for children it should be in diluted form (or another preparation should be used).

▲ side-effects: there is commonly skin irritation; there may also be a temporary burning sensation. Sensitivity may cause a rash.

✚ warning: keep Ascabiol away from the eyes, and avoid taking it by the mouth.

Ascalix (*Wallace*) is a proprietary non-prescription ANTHELMINTIC drug used to treat infestation by threadworms or roundworms. Produced in the form of syrup (in bottles and in sachets), Ascalix is a preparation of piperazine hydrate.

▲/✚ side-effects/warning: *see* PIPERAZINE.

Attenuvax (*Morson*) is a proprietary VACCINE against measles (rubeola), available only on prescription. It is a powdered preparation of live but weakened measles viruses for administration by injection. Attenuvax is not usually recommended for children aged under 12 months.

▲ side-effects: there may be inflammation at the site of injection. Rarely, there may be high temperature, a rash, swelling of the lymph glands and/or pain in the joints.

✚ warning: Attenuvax should not be administered to patients who suffer from any infection, particularly tuberculosis; who are allergic to chicken, chicken feathers or eggs (the viruses are cultured in chick-embryo tissue); who have known immune-system abnormalities; who are pregnant; or who are already taking corticosteroid drugs (except for replacement therapy), cytotoxic drugs or undergoing radiation treatment. It should be administered with caution to those who suffer from epilepsy or any other condition potentially involving convulsive fits. The vaccine contains NEOMYCIN, so should not be administered to those who are allergic to this drug.

Audicort (*Lederle*) is a proprietary anti-inflammatory ANTI-BACTERIAL and ANTIFUNGAL, available only on prescription, used in the treatment of bacterial and/or fungal infections of the outer ear. It contains the CORTICOSTEROID triamcinolone acetonide, the local anaesthetic benzocaine, the ANTIBIOTIC neomycin, and the ANTIFUNGAL drug undecenoic acid.

▲/✚ side-effects/warning: *see* NEOMYCIN.

Augmentin (*Beecham*) is a proprietary preparation of the penicillin-like ANTIBIOTIC amoxycillin together with an enhancing agent, clavulanic acid. This inhibits enzymes produced by some bacteria (penicillinases), which break down amoxycillin so making it ineffective. Thus the combination is active against many infections which would normally be resistant to amoxycillin alone. It extends the range and efficiency of amoxycillin as an antibiotic.

It is used primarily to treat infections of the skin, ear, nose and throat, and urinary tract, and is produced in a number of forms: as tablets, as a solution (under the name Augmentin Dispersible), in milder versions as a powder for solution (under the names Augmentin Paediatric and Augmentin Junior), and in vials for injections or infusion (under the trade name Augmentin Intravenous).
▲/✚ side-effects/warning: *see* AMOXYCILLIN.

Aureocort (*Lederle*) is a proprietary ANTIBIOTIC preparation for topical application, available only on prescription, used to treat inflammations of the skin where infection is also present. Produced as a water-miscible cream, an anhydrous ointment, and an aerosol spray, Aureocort contains the CORTICOSTEROID triamcinolone acetonide and the TETRACYCLINE antibiotic chlortetracycline hydrochloride.
▲/✚ side-effects/warning: *see* CHLORTETRACYCLINE.

Aureomycin (*Lederle*) is a proprietary broad-spectrum ANTIBIOTIC, available only on prescription, used to treat a wide range of bacterial infections. It is produced in the form of capsules (in which form it is not recommended for women who are pregnant or for children under 12 years), as a cream and as an ointment. In every form it is a preparation of the TETRACYCLINE chlortetracycline hydrochloride.
▲/✚ side-effects/warning: *see* CHLORTETRACYCLINE.

Avloclor (*ICI*) is a proprietary ANTIMALARIAL drug, available only on prescription, used primarily to prevent or treat certain forms of malaria, but also used as an AMOEBICIDAL drug to treat amoebic hepatitis, and to treat rheumatoid arthritis. Produced in the form of tablets, Avloclor is a preparation of chloroquine phosphate. In children under 12 years of age, Avloclor is used only to prevent or to suppress malaria.
▲/✚ side-effects/warning: *see* CHLOROQUINE.

Azactam (*Squibb*) is a proprietary ANTIBIOTIC, available only on prescription, used to treat severe infections caused by gram-negative bacteria, including gonorrhoea and infections of the urinary tract. Produced in the form of powder for reconstitution as a medium for injection or infusion, Azactam is a preparation of aztreonam.

▲/✚ side-effects/warning: *see* AZTREONAM.

azlocillin is a penicillin-type ANTIBIOTIC used primarily to treat infections by a type of gram-negative bacteria called Pseudomonas, and particularly in serious infections of the urinary tract and respiratory tract, and for septicaemia. Administration is by injection or infusion.

▲ side-effects: there may be some allergic reactions − such as a rash − and high temperature; some patients experience pain in the joints. Diarrhoea may occur.

✚ warning: azlocillin should not be administered to patients who are known to be allergic to penicillins; it should be administered with caution to those who have impaired kidney function, or who are pregnant.
Related article: SECUROPEN.

aztreonam is an ANTIBIOTIC used to treat severe infections caused by gram-negative bacteria. Administration is by injection or infusion. A relatively recent addition to the pharmacopoeia of the beta lactam type (which includes the penicillins), aztreonam is thought to arouse fewer sensitivity reactions than are caused by many other antibiotics of the beta lactam type.

▲ side-effects: there may be diarrhoea and vomiting; skin rashes may occur, with pain or inflammation at the site of injection or infusion. Rarely, there may be reduction in the number of white cells in the blood, causing bleeding and lowered resistance to infection.

✚ warning: aztreonam should not be administered to patients who are pregnant; it should be administered with caution to those who are known to be sensitive to penicillin or cephalosporin, who have impaired kidney or liver function, or who are lactating.
Related article: AZACTAM.

bacampicillin hydrochloride is a broad-spectrum penicillin-type ANTIBIOTIC, a derivative of AMPICILLIN that is converted to ampicillin in the bloodstream. Used to treat many infections, especially those of the urogenital areas, upper respiratory tract and middle ear, it is administered orally in the form of tablets.

▲ side-effects: there may be sensitivity reactions, ranging from a minor rash to urticaria, high temperature and joint pain, or even to anaphylactic shock. The most common side-effect, however, is simply diarrhoea.

✚ warning: bacampicillin hydrochloride should not be administered to patients who are known to be allergic to penicillin-type antibiotics; it should be administered with caution to those with impaired kidney function. *Related article:* AMBAXIN.

Bacticlens (*Smith & Nephew*) is a proprietary non-prescription DISINFECTANT, used to treat minor wounds and burns on the skin. Produced in the form of a solution in sachets, Bacticlens is a preparation of chlorhexidine gluconate.

▲/✚ side-effects/warning: *see* CHLORHEXIDINE.

Bactigras (*Smith & Nephew*) is a proprietary non-prescription dressing in the form of gauze impregnated with chlorhexidine acetate. It is used to treat wounds and ulcers.

▲/✚ side-effects/warning: *see* CHLORHEXIDINE.

Bactrian (*Loveridge*) is a proprietary non-prescription ANTISEPTIC cream used in the treatment of minor burns and abrasions. It contains the antiseptic CETRIMIDE in very dilute solution.

Bactrim (*Roche*) is a proprietary ANTIBACTERIAL available only on prescription, used to treat bacterial infections, especially infections of the urinary tract, sinusitis and bronchitis, and infections of bones and joints. Produced in the form of tablets (in three strengths), as soluble (dispersible) tablets, as a suspension for dilution (the

B

potency of the suspension once dilute is retained for 14 days), as a sugar-free syrup for dilution (the potency of the syrup once dilute is retained for 14 days), in ampoules for injection, and in ampoules for intravenous infusion (following dilution). Bactrim is a compound preparation, co-trimoxazole, which is five parts of a SULPHONAMIDE, sulphamethazole, to one part of TRIMETHOPRIM.
▲/✚ side-effects/warning: *see* CO-TRIMOXAZOLE.

Bactroban (*Beecham*) is a proprietary ANTIBIOTIC, available only on prescription, used in topical application to treat bacterial infections of the skin. Produced in the form of a water-miscible ointment, Bactroban is a preparation of mupirocin in dilute solution.
✚ warning: the ointment may sting on application.

Bactroban nasal (*Beecham*) is a proprietary ANTIBIOTIC available only on prescription, used to treat staphylococcal infections in and around the nostrils. Produced in the form of an ointment for topical application, Bactroban nasal is a preparation of the antibiotic drug mupirocin.
▲/✚ side-effects/warning: *see* MUPIROCIN.

Banocide (*Wellcome*) is a proprietary preparation of the drug diethylcarbamazine, used to treat infestations by filarial worm-parasites (such as those that cause elephantiasis, lymphangitis, loiasis and onchocerciasis). It may also be used to treat certain stages of toxocaral infections. Side-effects are inevitable, and may be severe (but should be treated with other drugs); close monitoring is essential throughout treatment, but particularly at first. Several courses of treatment may be necessary. It is produced in the form of tablets.
▲/✚ side-effects/warning: *see* DIETHYLCARBAMAZINE.

Barquinol HC (*Fisons*) is a proprietary non-prescription corticosteroid cream used to treat mild inflammations of the skin. Apart from its anti-inflammatory properties it also has some ANTIBACTERIAL and ANTIFUNGAL activity

because in addition to the steroid hydrocortisone acetate it also contains the iodine-based antiseptic clioquinol.
▲/✚ side-effects/warning: *see* CLIOQUINOL.

B

Baxan (*Bristol-Myers*) is a proprietary ANTIBIOTIC, available only on prescription, used to treat many infections, especially those of the skin and soft tissues, the respiratory and urinary tracts, and the middle ear. Produced in the form of capsules, and as a suspension (in three strengths) for dilution, Baxan is a preparation of the CEPHALOSPORIN cefadroxil monohydrate.
▲/✚ side-effects/warning: *see* CEFADROXIL.

Baypen (*Bayer*) is a proprietary broad-spectrum penicillin-type ANTIBIOTIC, used to treat many infections and to prevent others following abdominal and/or uterine surgery. Produced in the form of powder in vials for reconstitution as a medium for injection or infusion, Baypen is a preparation of mezlocillin.
▲/✚ side-effects/warning: *see* MEZLOCILLIN.

BCG vaccine (*bacillus Calmette-Guérin* vaccine) is a strain of the tuberculosis bacillus that no longer causes the disease in humans but does cause the formation in the body of the specific antibodies, and so can be used as the base for an ANTITUBERCULAR vaccine. It is administered intradermally.

benethamine penicillin is a penicillin-type ANTIBIOTIC that is used, along with other penicillins, to treat and prevent infections caused by sensitive gram-positive organisms such as streptococci. It is a very soluble salt of BENZYLPENICILLIN (penicillin G), which is slowly released from the injection site to give low plasma levels over a long period of time. Administration is by deep intramuscular injection.
▲ side-effects: there may be sensitivity reactions ranging from a minor rash to urticaria and joint pains, and (occasionally) to high temperature or anaphylactic shock.

21

B

✚ warning: benethamine penicillin should not be administered to patients who are known to be allergic to penicillins; it should be administered with caution to those who suffer from impaired kidney function.
Related articles: CAPITOL; TRIPLOPEN.

benzalkonium chloride is an astringent ANTISEPTIC that also has some keratolytic properties and may be used in topical application to remove hard, dead skin from around wounds or ulcers, or to dissolve warts. It is also used on minor abrasions and burns, and (in the form of lozenges to be sucked) on mouth ulcers or gum disease, simply as a disinfectant. For other than oral purposes, administration is topical in the form of a cream or, combined with bromine, as a paint.
✚ warning: in topical application, keep benzalkonium chloride off normal skin.
Related articles: CAPITOL; DRAPOLENE.

benzathine penicillin is a penicillin-type ANTIBIOTIC that is used to treat many bacterial infections. In high dosage, given intramuscularly, it is used especially to treat syphilis (although PROCAINE PENICILLIN appears more effective in this) or to prevent patients at risk from contracting rheumatic fever. Administration is oral in the form of a suspension or drops, or by injection.
▲ side-effects: there may be sensitivity reactions ranging from a minor rash to urticaria and joint pains, and (occasionally) to high temperature or anaphylactic shock.
✚ warning: benzathine penicillin should not be administered to patients who are known to be allergic to penicillins; it should be administered with caution to those with impaired kidney function.
Related article: PENIDURAL.

benzoic acid ointment is a non-proprietary ANTIFUNGAL compound formulation (known also as Whitfield's ointment) used most commonly to treat patches of the fungal infection ringworm. It contains the active substances benzoic acid and salicylic acid in an emulsifying ointment base.

benzyl benzoate is a transparent liquid with an aromatic smell, used to treat infestation of the skin of the trunk and limbs by itch-mites (scabies) or by lice (pediculosis). A skin irritant, it is not suitable for use on the head, face and neck, and treatment of children should be in diluted form (or by another preparation altogether). Administration is in the form of a from-the-neck-down application two days consecutively, without washing in the interval.
Related article: ASCABIOL.

benzylpenicillin is the chemical name for the first of the penicillins to be isolated and used as an ANTIBIOTIC. An alternative name is penicillin G. Despite the many hundreds of antibiotics introduced since, it still remains the drug of choice in treating many severe infections including those caused by sensitive strains of meningococcus (meningitis, septicaemia), pneumococcus (pneumonia, meningitis) and streptococcus (bacterial sore throat, scarlet fever, septicaemia). In its long-acting forms, PROCAINE PENICILLIN and BENZATHINE PENICILLIN, it has an important role in treating gonorrhea and syphilis. Since benzylpenicillin is inactivated by digestive acids in the stomach it has to be injected. Its rapid excretion by the kidney also means frequent administration is necessary, unless long-acting preparations are used.
▲ side-effects: there may be sensitivity reactions ranging from a minor rash to urticaria and joint pains, and (occasionally) to high temperature or anaphylactic shock.
✚ warning: benzylpenicillin should not be administered to patients known to be allergic to penicillins; it should be administered with caution to those with impaired kidney function.
Related article: CRYSTAPEN.

bephenium is an ANTHELMINTIC drug used specifically to treat infestation of the small intestine by hookworms,

B

which draw blood from the point of their attachment to the intestinal wall and may thus cause iron-deficiency anaemia. Administration is oral in the form of a solution.

▲ side-effects: there may be occasional nausea and vomiting; some patients experience diarrhoea, headache and vertigo.

Related article: ALCOPAR.

Berkmycen (*Berk*) is a proprietary ANTIBIOTIC, available only on prescription, used to treat infections of the soft tissues and respiratory tract. Produced in the form of tablets, Berkmycen is a preparation of the TETRACYCLINE oxytetracycline dihydrate. It should not be used for children aged under 2 years.

▲/✚ side-effects/warning: *see* OXYTETRACYCLINE.

Betadine (*Napp*) is a proprietary non-prescription group of preparations of the ANTISEPTIC povidone-iodine, produced in the form of pessaries, a gel and a solution (all together a vaginal cleansing kit) for the treatment of bacterial infections in the vagina and cervix. A more dilute solution may also be used as a mouthwash and gargle for inflammations in the mouth and throat. For the treatment of skin infections it is produced in solutions of differing concentrations as an aerosol spray, an antiseptic paint, an alcoholic lotion, a scalp and skin cleanser, a shampoo, a skin cleanser solution, and a surgical scrub; it is also produced as a dry powder for insufflation. In the form of a water-miscible ointment it is used to dress leg ulcers.

▲/✚ side-effects/warning: *see* POVIDONE-IODINE.

Bilarcil is a preparation of the organo-phosphorous drug METRIPHONATE, used specifically to treat infections by parasitic *Schistosoma haematobium* worms (which cause bilharziasis) in various organs. It is not marketed in the United Kingdom.

Bocasan (*Cooper*) is a proprietary non-prescription ANTISEPTIC, used to cleanse and disinfect the mouth.

Produced in the form of sealed sachets to be emptied into water to produce a mouth-wash, Bocasin is a preparation of sodium perborate.

✚ warning: see SODIUM PERBORATE.

botulism antitoxin is a preparation that neutralizes the toxins produced by the botulism bacteria (rather than acting to counter the presence of the bacteria, as would a vaccine). In this way, it may be administered not only to people at risk from the disease following exposure to an infected patient, but also to the infected patient as a means of treatment. However, there are some strains of botulism in relation to which the antitoxin is not effective. Moreover, hypersensitivity reactions are common (and it is essential that an administering doctor has all relevant details of a patient's medical history, with regard especially to allergies). Administration is by injection or infusion, depending on whether it is for the purpose of prophylaxis or treatment.

Bradosol (*Ciba*) is a proprietary non-prescription DISINFECTANT, used to treat infections in the mouth and throat. Produced in the form of lozenges, Bradosol is a preparation of the detergent antiseptic domiphen bromide.

brilliant green and crystal violet paint is a non-proprietary antiseptic paint used primarily to prepare skin for surgery. It combines the two dyes brilliant green and gentian violet (also called crystal violet).
see GENTIAN VIOLET.

Britcin (*DDSA Pharmaceuticals*) is a proprietary ANTIBIOTIC, available only on prescription, used to treat systemic bacterial infections and infections of the upper respiratory tract, of the ear, nose and throat, and of the urogenital areas. Produced in the form of capsules (in two strengths), Britcin is a preparation of the broad-spectrum PENICILLIN ampicillin.

▲/✚ side-effects/warning: *see* AMPICILLIN.

B

B

Brolene (*May & Baker*) is a proprietary non-prescription preparation with ANTIFUNGAL and ANTIBACTERIAL properties, used to treat bacterial infections in the eyelid and conjunctiva. Produced in the form of eye-drops, Brolene is a preparation of propamidine isethionate.

Broxil (*Beecham*) is a proprietary ANTIBIOTIC, available only on prescription, used to treat many forms of infection, in particular streptococcal infections of the throat, middle ear and skin. Produced in the form of capsules, and as a syrup for dilution (the potency of the syrup once dilute is retained for 7 days), Broxil is a preparation of the PENICILLIN derivative phenethicillin.
▲/✚ side-effects/warning: *see* PHENETHICILLIN.

calcium sulphaloxate is a SULPHONAMIDE that has now largely been replaced by others because it is poorly absorbed. Formerly, however, it was popularly prescribed to treat infections of the intestines and to prevent infection during surgery. It is still sometimes used to treat chronic diarrhoea. Use may lead to the appearance of rashes.

Calthor (*Ayerst*) is a proprietary broad-spectrum ANTIBIOTIC of the penicillin family, available only on prescription, used to treat bronchitis and infections of the soft tissues and urinary tract. Produced in the form of tablets (in two strengths) and as a syrup for dilution, Calthor is a preparation of ciclacillin. Calthor is not recommended for children aged under 2 months.
✚ warning: *see* CICLACILLIN.

Canesten (*Bayer*) is a proprietary non-prescription ANTIFUNGAL preparation, used to treat particularly vaginal thrush and dermatophyte infections of the skin, such as athlete's foot. Treatment is topical and should be continued for the full course to prevent recurrence. Produced in the form of vaginal tablets (pessaries), as a solution, as a spray, as a cream and as a dusting-powder, Canesten is a preparation of clotrimazole. Canesten vaginal cream, vaginal tablets (in two strengths) and a Duopak containing vaginal tablets and cream are available only on prescription.
▲/✚ side-effects/warning: *see* CLOTRIMAZOLE.

Canesten 1 (*Bayer*) is a proprietary ANTIFUNGAL preparation, available only on prescription, used to treat vaginal infections. Produced in the form of vaginal tablets (pessaries), Canesten 1 − which is a stronger version of CANESTEN − is also a preparation of clotrimazole.
▲/✚ side-effects/warning: *see* CLOTRIMAZOLE.

Canesten 10% VC (*Bayer*) is a proprietary ANTIFUNGAL cream, available only on prescription, used to treat vaginal infections. To be inserted through a special

27

applicator, Canesten 10% VC is a preparation of clotrimazole.

▲/✚ side-effects/warning: *see* CLOTRIMAZOLE.

Canesten-HC (*Bayer*) is a proprietary ANTIFUNGAL CORTICOSTEROID preparation, available only on prescription, used to treat fungal infections, particularly those that cause inflammation. Produced in the form of a cream for topical application, Canesten-HC consists of a combination of clotrimazole and hydrocortisone.

▲/✚ side-effects/warning: *see* CLOTRIMAZOLE.

Capastat (*Dista*) is a proprietary ANTITUBERCULAR drug, used to treat tuberculosis resistant to other drugs. Produced in the form of powder for reconstitution as intramuscular injections, Capastat is a preparation of the ANTIBIOTIC capreomycin sulphate. It is not usually recommended for children.

▲/✚ side-effects/warning: *see* CAPREOMYCIN.

Capitol (*Dermal*) is a proprietary non-prescription ANTIBACTERIAL preparation, used to treat dandruff and other scalp conditions. Produced in the form of a gel applied as a shampoo, Capitol is a preparation of the antiseptic BENZALKONIUM CHLORIDE.

capreomycin is an ANTIBIOTIC drug used specifically in the treatment of tuberculosis that proves to be resistant to the first-line drugs, or in cases where those drugs are not tolerated. Administration is by intramuscular injection.

✚ warning: capreomycin should not be administered to patients who are pregnant, and should be administered with caution to those who have impaired function of the liver, kidney or sense of hearing (functions that should be monitored during treatment), or who are already taking other ototoxic antibiotics, or who are lactating.

▲ side-effects: there may be kidney toxicity and impaired hearing with or without ringing in the ears (tinnitus)

or vertigo; sometimes there are sensitivity reactions such as rashes or urticaria.
Related article: CAPASTAT

C

carbaryl is an insecticide used in the treatment of scalp or pubic lice. Administration is (in aqueous or alcohol solution) in the form of a lotion, or shampoo which is applied to wet hair, allowed to dry, and then rinsed after a specified time (usually about 12 hours). The procedure may need to be repeated after a week.
✚ warning: keep away from the eyes.
Related articles: CARYLDERM; CLINICIDE; DERBAC-C; SULEO-C.

carbenicillin is an ANTIBIOTIC of the penicillin family. Used to treat serious infections caused by sensitive gram-negative organisms, often in combination with aminoglycoside antibiotics. Administration is by injection or infusion in the case of systemic infections, or by intramuscular injections for urinary tract infections. It has now largely been superseded by more potent agents.
▲ side-effects: there may be sensitivity reactions – serious ones in hypersensitive patients. Body temperature may rise, and there may be pains in the joints and skin rashes or urticaria; potassium and platelet levels in the blood may decline.
✚ warning: carbenicillin should not be administered to patients known to be sensitive to penicillins, and should be administered with caution to those who suffer from impaired kidney function.
Related article: PYOPEN.

carfecillin sodium is a penicillin-like ANTIBIOTIC with a similar spectrum of activity to CARBENICILLIN. It is used particularly to treat susceptible gram-negative infections of the urinary tract. Administration is oral in the form of tablets.
▲ side-effects: there may be sensitivity reactions – serious ones in hypersensitive patients. Body temperature may rise, and there may be pains in the joints and skin rashes or urticaria.

✚ warning: carfecillin sodium should not be administered to patients known to be sensitive to penicillin, and should be administered with caution to those with impaired kidney function.
Related article: UTICILLIN.

Carylderm (*Napp*) is a proprietary non-prescription drug used to treat infestations of the scalp and pubic hair by lice. Produced in the form of a lotion and a shampoo, Carylderm is a preparation of the pediculicide carbaryl.
✚ warning: see CARBARYL.

cefaclor is a broad-spectrum ANTIBIOTIC, one of the first generation CEPHALOSPORINS, now primarily used to treat infections of the urinary tract and the respiratory tract. Administration is oral in the form of capsules or a dilute suspension.
▲ side-effects: there may be sensitivity reactions − some of which may be serious. Sometimes there is nausea and vomiting, with diarrhoea.
✚ warning: cefaclor should not be administered to patients who might be sensitive to penicillins in general and cephalosporins in particular. It should be administered with caution to those with impaired kidney function. Prolonged skin reactions may occur in children.
Related article: DISTACLOR.

cefadroxil is a broad-spectrum ANTIBIOTIC, one of the first generation CEPHALOSPORINS, now primarily used to treat bacterial infections of the skin, soft tissues and the urinary tract. Administration is oral in the form of capsules or a dilute suspension.
▲ side-effects: there may be sensitivity reactions − some of which may be serious. Sometimes there is nausea and vomiting, with diarrhoea.
✚ warning: cefadroxil should not be administered to patients who might be sensitive to penicillins in general and cephalosporins in particular. It should be

administered with caution to those who suffer from impaired kidney function.

Related article: BAXAN.

Cefizox (*Wellcome*) is a proprietary ANTIBIOTIC, available only on prescription, used to treat gonorrhoea and infections in the upper respiratory tract and urinary tract. Produced in the form of powder for reconstitution as injections, Cefizox is a preparation of the CEPHALOSPORIN ceftizoxime as a salt of sodium. It is not recommended for children aged under 3 months.

▲/✚ side-effects/warning: *see* CEFTIZOXIME.

cefotaxime is a broad-spectrum ANTIBIOTIC, one of the third generation CEPHALOSPORINS, used to treat a wide range of bacterial infections, particularly of the skin and soft tissues, the urinary tract, the meninges of the brain (meningitis) and the blood (septicaemia). It is also used to prevent infection during surgery. Administration is by intravenous or intramuscular injection.

▲ side-effects: there may be sensitivity reactions − some of which may be serious. Sometimes there is nausea and vomiting, with diarrhoea.

✚ warning: cefotaxime should not be administered to patients who might be sensitive to penicillins in general and cephalosporins in particular. It should be administered with caution to those with impaired kidney function, or who are pregnant or lactating.

Related article: CLAFORAN.

cefoxitin is a broad-spectrum ANTIBIOTIC, one of the second generation CEPHALOSPORINS, used to treat a wide range of bacterial infections, particularly gram-negative infections of the skin and soft tissues, the urinary tract, the respiratory tract, the peritoneum (peritonitis) and the blood (septicaemia). Because of its activity against mixed aerobic and anaerobic *Bacteroides fragilis* infections it is also used to prevent infection during or following gynaecological or obstetric surgery. Administration is by intravenous or intramuscular injection.

▲ side-effects: there may be sensitivity reactions − some of which may be serious. Sometimes there is nausea and vomiting, with diarrhoea.

✚ warning: cefoxitin should not be administered to patients who might be sensitive to penicillins in general and cephalosporins in particular. It should be administered with caution to those with impaired kidney function.

Related article: MEFOXIN.

cefsulodin is a broad-spectrum ANTIBIOTIC, one of the first generation CEPHALOSPORINS, used primarily to treat pseudomonal infections and for surgical prophylaxis. Administration is by intravenous or intramuscular injection.

▲ side-effects: there may be sensitivity reactions − some of which may be serious. Sometimes there is nausea and vomiting, with diarrhoea.

✚ warning: cefsulodin should not be administered to patients who might be sensitive to penicillins in general and cephalosporins in particular. It should be administered with caution to those with impaired kidney function, or who are pregnant. Monitoring of blood counts during treatment is essential.

Related article: MONASPOR.

ceftazidime is a broad-spectrum ANTIBIOTIC, one of the third generation CEPHALOSPORINS. It is the most active of the cephalosporins against bacterial infections, particularly of the skin and soft tissues, the urinary tract, the respiratory tract, the ear, nose and throat, the bones and the joints, the gastrointestinal tract, the meninges (meningitis) and the blood (septicaemia). It is also used to treat infection in patients whose immune systems are defective. Administration is by intravenous or intramuscular injection.

▲ side-effects: there may be sensitivity reactions − some of which may be serious. Alternatively, sometimes there is nausea and vomiting, with diarrhoea.

✚ warning: ceftazidime should not be administered to

patients who might be sensitive to penicillins in general and cephalosporins in particular, or to patients who are already taking certain diuretic drugs. It should be administered with caution to those who suffer from impaired kidney function, or who are pregnant.
Related article: FORTUM.

C

ceftizoxime is a broad-spectrum ANTIBIOTIC, one of the third generation CEPHALOSPORINS, used to treat a wide range of gram-negative bacterial infections, particularly of the skin and soft tissues, the urinary tract, the genital organs, the lower respiratory tract, the meninges of the brain (meningitis) and the blood (septicaemia). It is also used to treat infection in patients whose immune systems are defective. Administration is by intravenous or intramuscular injection.
▲ side-effects: there may be sensitivity reactions − some of which may be serious. Alternatively, sometimes there is nausea and vomiting, with diarrhoea.
✚ warning: ceftizoxime should not be administered to patients who might be sensitive to penicillins in general and cephalosporins in particular. It should be administered with caution to those who suffer from impaired kidney function.
Related article: CEFIZOX.

cefuroxime is a broad-spectrum ANTIBIOTIC, one of the second generation CEPHALOSPORINS, used to treat a wide range of bacterial infections, particularly gram-negative infections of the urinary tract, the respiratory tract, the genital tract, and the meninges (meningitis). It is also used to prevent infection during surgery. Administration is by intravenous or intramuscular injection.
▲ side-effects: there may be sensitivity reactions − some of which may be serious. Alternatively, sometimes there is nausea and vomiting, with diarrhoea.
✚ warning: cefuroxime should not be administered to patients who might be sensitive to penicillins in general and cephalosporins in particular, or to patients who are already taking certain diuretic drugs. It

should be administered with caution to those who suffer from impaired kidney function, or who are pregnant.
Related article: ZINACEF.

Celbenin (*Beecham*) is a proprietary penicillin-type ANTIBIOTIC, available only on prescription, used to treat many forms of infection but particularly those caused by penicillin-resistant bacteria. Produced in the form of powder for reconstitution as injections, Celbenin is a preparation of methicillin sodium.
▲/✚ side-effects/warning: *see* METHICILLIN.

cephalexin is a broad-spectrum ANTIBIOTIC, one of the orally active CEPHALOSPORINS, which may be used to treat a wide range of bacterial infections, particularly sensitive urinary tract infections. Administration is in the form of capsules, tablets and liquids.
▲ side-effects: there may be sensitivity reactions — some of which may be serious. Sometimes there is nausea and vomiting, with diarrhoea.
✚ warning: cephalexin should not be administered to patients who might be sensitive to penicillins in general and cephalosporins in particular. It should be administered with caution to those with impaired kidney function.
Related articles: CEPOREX; KEFLEX.

cephalosporins are broad-spectrum ANTIBIOTICS that act against both gram-positive and gram-negative bacteria. They bear a strong resemblance in chemical structure to the penicillins: both contain a beta lactam ring, hence their classification as beta lactam antibiotics. The similarity in structure extends to mechanism of action: both inhibit the synthesis of the bacterial cell wall, so killing growing bacteria (bactericidal). As a group the cephalosporins are generally active against streptococci, staphylococci and a number of gram-negative bacteria including many coliforms. Some second generation cephalosporins are resistant to inactivation by bacterial pencillinase enzymes; this widens the range of sensitive gram-negative organisms, including *Haemophilus influenzae.* Some of the latest, third generation, cephalosporins, such as ceftazidime, are active against pseudomonal infections. Many cephalosporins are actively excreted by the kidney, therefore reaching considerably higher concentrations in the urine than in the blood. For this reason they may be used to treat infections of the urinary tract during their own excretion. In general cephalosporins are rarely the drug of first choice, but provide a useful alternative or reserve option for particular situations. The currently used cephalosporins are relatively non-toxic, with only occasional blood clotting problems, superinfections and hypersensitivity reactions (only 10% of patients allergic to penicillin show sensitivity to cephalosporins).

▲/✚ side-effects/warning: *see* CEFACLOR; CEFADROXIL; CEFOTAXIME; CEFOXITIN; CEFSULODIN; CEFTAZIDIME; CEFTIZOXIME; CEFUROXIME; CEPHALEXIN; CEPHALOTHIN; CEPHAMANDOLE; CEPHAZOLIN; CEPHRADINE; LATAMOXEF DISODIUM.

cephalothin is a broad-spectrum ANTIBIOTIC, one of the first CEPHALOSPORINS, which can be used to treat a wide range of bacterial infections, particularly of the skin and soft tissues, the urinary tract, upper respiratory tract, and middle ear. It is also used to prevent infection during surgery. Administration is by injection.

▲ side-effects: there may be sensitivity reactions – some of which may be serious. Sometimes there is nausea and vomiting, with diarrhoea.

✚ warning: cephalothin should not be administered to patients who might be sensitive to penicillins in general and cephalosporins in particular, or to those with impaired kidney functions.

Related article: KEFLIN.

cephamandole is a broad-spectrum ANTIBIOTIC, one of the second generation CEPHALOSPORINS. It is less susceptible to inactivation by bacterial penicillinases, and for this reason is effective against a greater range of gram-negative bacteria such as penicillin resistant *Neisseria gonorrhoeae* and *Haemophilus influenzae*. Cephamandole is used to treat a wide range of bacterial infections, particularly of the skin and soft tissues, the genito-urinary tract, upper respiratory tract, and middle ear. It is also used to prevent infection during surgery. Administration is by injection.

▲ side-effects: there may be sensitivity reactions − some of which may be serious. Sometimes there is nausea and vomiting, with diarrhoea.

✚ warning: cephamandole should not be administered to patients who might be sensitive to penicillins in general and cephalosporins in particular. It should be administered with caution to those with impaired kidney function.

Related article: KEFADOL.

cephazolin is a broad-spectrum ANTIBIOTIC, one of the first CEPHALOSPORINS, used to treat a wide range of bacterial infections, particularly of the skin and soft tissues, urinary tract, upper respiratory tract, and middle ear. It is also used to prevent infection during surgery. Administration is by injection.

▲ side-effects: there may be sensitivity reactions − some of which may be serious. Sometimes there is nausea and vomiting, with diarrhoea.

✚ warning: cephazolin should not be administered to patients who might be sensitive to penicillins in general and cephalosporins in particular. It should be administered with caution to those with impaired kidney function.

Related article: KEFZOL.

cephradine is a broad-spectrum ANTIBIOTIC, one of the first CEPHALOSPORINS, used to treat a wide range of bacterial infections, particularly streptococcal infections of the skin and soft tissues, the urinary tract, upper respiratory tract, and middle ear. It is also used to prevent infection during surgery. Administration is oral in the form of capsules or a dilute syrup, or by injection.

▲ side-effects: there may be sensitivity reactions — some of which may be serious. Sometimes there is nausea and vomiting, with diarrhoea.

✚ warning: cephradine should not be administered to patients who might be sensitive to penicillins in general and cephalosporins in particular. It should be administered with caution to those with impaired kidney function.

Related article: VELOSEF.

Ceporex (*Glaxo*) is a proprietary ANTIBIOTIC, available only on prescription, used to treat infections in the respiratory tract, urogenital area, soft tissues and middle ear. Produced in the form of capsules (in two strengths), as tablets (in two strengths), as drops for children, as a suspension (in two strengths), and as a syrup (in three strengths) for dilution (the potency of the syrup once diluted is retained for 7 days), Ceporex is a preparation of the CEPHALOSPORIN cephalexin.

▲/✚ side-effects/warning: *see* CEPHALEXIN.

Cetavlex (*Care*) is a proprietary non-prescription ANTISEPTIC, used to treat cuts and abrasions. Produced in the form of a water-based cream, Cetavlex's active constituent is CETRIMIDE.

Cetavlon (*ICI*) is a proprietary non-prescription DISINFECTANT, used to treat skin and scalp conditions, or in cleansing cuts and burns. Produced in the form of a solution, Cetavlon's active constituent is CETRIMIDE.

Cetriclens (*Smith & Nephew Medical*) is a proprietary non-prescription DISINFECTANT, used to clean skin and wounds. Produced in the form of a solution (in two strengths, the stronger under the name Cetriclens Forte), Cetriclens is a compound preparation of two antiseptics, CHLORHEXIDINE gluconate and CETRIMIDE.

cetrimide is a detergent that has ANTISEPTIC properties; therapeutically, it is often combined with the antiseptic

CHLORHEXIDINE. It is used in the form of a solution as a disinfectant for the skin and scalp, burns and wounds and in the form of a water-miscible cream as a soap substitute in the care of conditions such as acne and seborrhoea. In use, it should be kept away from the eyes and out of body cavities; some patients find it a mild skin irritant.

Chemotrim Paed (*RP Drugs*) is a proprietary ANTIBIOTIC, available only on prescription, used to treat infections of the respiratory, urinary and gastrointestinal tracts. Produced in the form of a suspension specifically intended for children, Chemotrim Paed is a compound combination of the SULPHONAMIDE sulphamethoxazole with trimethoprim — a compound itself known as co-trimoxazole. It is not recommended for children aged under 6 weeks.

▲/✚ side-effects/warning: *see* CO-TRIMOXAZOLE; SULPHAMETHOXAZOLE; TRIMETHOPRIM.

chloramphenicol is a broad-spectrum ANTIBIOTIC with the capacity to treat many forms of infection effectively. However, the serious side-effects that accompany its systemic use demand that it is ordinarily restricted to the treatment of certain severe infections such as typhoid fever, haemophilus meningitis and some other penicillin-resistant forms of meningitis. In topical application to the eyes, ears or skin, when its serious toxicity is not encountered, the drug is useful in treating such conditions as bacterial conjunctivitis, otitis externa, or many types of skin infection. Topical administration is in the form of eye-drops, ear-drops or a cream. Systemic administration is in the form of capsules or a dilute suspension, or by injection or infusion.

▲ side-effects: idiosyncratic reactions are rare, but potentially life-threatening. Systemic treatment may cause serious damage to the bone marrow, resulting in critical blood cell deficiencies

✚ warning: chloramphenicol should not be administered to patients who are pregnant or lactating; it should be administered with caution to those with impaired liver or kidney function. In forms for topical application, it should be kept away from open wounds. Prolonged or repeated use should be avoided. Regular blood counts are essential.

Related articles: CHLOROMYCETIN; KEMICETINE; MINIMS; OPULETS; SNO PHENICOL.

Chlorasept 2000 (*Travenol*) is a proprietary DISINFECTANT, available only on prescription, used to cleanse skin and wounds. Produced in sachets of solution (in five strengths), Chlorasept 2000 is a preparation of CHLORHEXIDINE acetate.

Chlorasol (*Schering-Prebbles*) is a proprietary non-prescription DISINFECTANT and cleanser, used to treat skin infections, and especially in cleansing wounds and ulcers. Produced in the form of a solution in sachets, Chlorasol is a preparation of SODIUM HYPOCHLORITE.

chlorhexidine is an ANTISEPTIC that is a constituent in many DISINFECTANT preparations, for use especially prior to surgery or in obstetrics, but that is primarily used (in the form of chlorhexidine gluconate, chlorhexidine acetate or chlorhexidine hydrochloride) either as a mouth wash for oral hygiene, or as a dressing for minor skin wounds and infections; it is also used for instillation in the bladder to relieve minor infections.

▲ side-effects: some patients experience sensitivity reactions.

✚ warning: caution should be exercised in assessing suitable solution concentration for bladder instillation: too high a concentration may lead to the appearance of blood in the urine. Avoid contact with mucous membranes.

Related articles: BACTICLENS; BACTIGRAS; CETRICLENS; CHLORASEPT 2000; CORSODYL; DISPRAY 1 QUICK PREP; ELUDRIL; HIBIDIL; HIBISCRUB; HIBISOL; HIBITANE; INSTILLAGEL; NASEPTIN; NYSTAFORM; ROTERSEPT; SAVLOCLENS; SAVLODIL; SAVLON HOSPITAL CONCENTRATE; TISEPT; TRAVASEPT; UNISEPT; UROTAINER.

chlorinated lime and boric acid solution is a non-proprietary formulation of chlorinated lime and boric acid, designed for topical application to disinfect and cleanse wounds and ulcers. It is applied as a wet dressing.

chlorinated soda solution is a non-proprietary formulation designed for topical application to disinfect and cleanse wounds and ulcers. Containing boric acid, chlorinated lime and sodium carbonate it is an irritant solution and surrounding tissues should be protected with a layer of petroleum jelly during treatment.

Chloromycetin (*Parke-Davis*) is a proprietary broad-spectrum ANTIBIOTIC, available only on prescription, used to treat potentially dangerous bacterial infections, such as typhoid fever and meningitis. Produced in the form of capsules, as a suspension for dilution (the potency of the dilute suspension is retained for 14 days), as eye-ointment and eye-drops, as a powder, and in vials for injection, Chloromycetin is a preparation of chloramphenicol.
▲/✚ side-effects/warning: *see* CHLORAMPHENICOL.

Chloromycetin Hydrocortisone (*Parke-Davis*) is a proprietary ANTIBIOTIC and CORTICOSTEROID preparation, available only on prescription, used to treat eye infections. Produced in the form of an eye ointment, Chloromycetin Hydrocortisone contains the antibiotic chloramphenicol and the steroid hydrocortisone.
▲/✚ side-effects/warning: *see* CHLORAMPHENICOL.

chloroquine is the major ANTIMALARIAL drug in use, effective against all three *Plasmodium* species that cause malaria, and used both to treat and to prevent contraction of the disease. However, it does not kill those forms of the parasite that migrate to the liver, and thus cannot prevent relapses caused by any form of *Plasmodium* that does so. Moreover, strains of *Plasmodium falciparum* have recently exhibited resistance to chloroquine in certain areas of the world, and in those areas alternative therapy is now advised.

Chloroquine is sometimes also used to treat infection
caused by amoebae, or to halt the progress of rheumatic
disease. Administration is oral in the form of tablets or a
dilute syrup, or by injection or infusion.

▲ side-effects: there may be nausea and vomiting, with
headache and itching; gastrointestinal disturbance may
be severe; some patients break out in a rash. Susceptible
patients may undergo psychotic episodes. Prolonged
high dosage may cause ringing in the ears (tinnitus) and
damage to the cornea and retina of the eyes.

✚ warning: chloroquine should not be administered to
patients with retinal disease, or who are allergic to
quinine; it should be administered with caution to
patients with porphyria, psoriasis, or who have
impaired kidney or liver function; who are elderly; or
who are children. Prolonged treatment should be
punctuated by ophthalmic checks.
Related articles: AVLOCLOR; MALARIVON; NIVAQUINE.

chloroxylenol is an ANTISEPTIC effective in killing some
bacteria but not others, and is an established constituent
in at least one well-known skin disinfectant. A few
patients experience mild skin irritation that may lead to
sensitivity reactions, however.
Related article: DETTOL.

chlortetracycline is a broad-spectrum TETRACYCLINE
ANTIBIOTIC used to treat many forms of infection caused
by several types of micro-organism; conditions it is
particularly used to treat include infections of the
urinary tract, of the respiratory tract, in and around the
eye, of the genital organs, and of the skin, including acne
and impetigo. Administration (as chlortetracycline
hydrochloride) is oral in the form of capsules or a
solution, or topical in the form of a cream, an ointment,
and an ophthalmic ointment.

▲ side-effects: there may be nausea and vomiting, with
diarrhoea. Occasionally, there is sensitivity to light or
some other sensitivity reaction.

✚ warning: chlortetracycline should not be administered

systemically to patients who are aged under 12 years, who are pregnant, or with impaired kidney function; it should be administered with caution to those who are lactating. The cream and the ointment may stain fabric.

Related article: AUREOMYCIN.

cholera vaccine is a suspension containing non-infective strains of the bacteria that causes cholera, a water- and food-borne disease that causes outbreaks of life-threatening vomiting and diarrhoea. Administration is initially by subcutaneous or intramuscular injection, followed 2 to 4 weeks later by a booster shot. The vaccine cannot guarantee total protection, and travellers should be warned still to take great care over the hygiene of the food and drink they consume. In any case, what protection is afforded lasts only for about 6 months.

Chymocyclar (*Armour*) is a proprietary tetracycline ANTIBIOTIC, available only on prescription, used to treat many forms of infection. Produced in the form of capsules, Chymocyclar contains tetracycline hydrochloride and the pancreatic enzymes trypsin and chymotrypsin. It is not recommended for children.

▲/✚ side-effects/warning: *see* TETRACYCLINE.

Cicatrin (*Calmic*) is a proprietary ANTIBIOTIC drug, available only on prescription, used by topical application to treat skin infections. Produced in the form of a cream, as a dusting-powder and as an aerosol powder-spray, Cicatrin's major active constituents include the antibiotics neomycin sulphate and bacitracin zinc.

▲/✚ side-effects/warning: *see* NEOMYCIN.

ciclacillin is an ANTIBIOTIC, a PENICILLIN derivative of ampicillin, used to treat infections of the upper respiratory tract, of the urinary tract, and of the soft tissues. Administration is oral in the form of tablets or a dilute suspension.

✚ warning: ciclacillin should not be administered to

patients known to be allergic to penicillins; it should be administered with caution to those with impaired kidney function.

▲ side-effects: the drug may cause diarrhoea if given in tablet form; there may be sensitivity reactions ranging from a minor rash to urticaria and joint pains, fever or anaphylactic shock.

Related article: CALTHOR.

Cidomycin (*Roussel*) is a proprietary ANTIBIOTIC, available only on prescription, used to treat many forms of infection, particularly serious gram-negative ones. Produced in ampoules for injection (in two strengths), in vials for the treatment of children, in ampoules for intrathecal injections, as a powder for reconstitution as a medium for injection, as ear- and eye-drops, as an eye ointment, and as a cream and an ointment for topical application, Cidomycin is a preparation of the aminoglycoside gentamicin sulphate.

▲/✚ side-effects/warning: *see* GENTAMICIN.

Cidomycin Topical (*Roussel*) is a proprietary ANTIBIOTIC preparation, available only on prescription, used in topical application to treat skin infections. Produced in the form of a water-miscible cream and a paraffin-based ointment, Cidomycin Topical is a preparation of the aminoglycoside gentamicin sulphate.

✚ warning: *see* GENTAMICIN.

Cinobac (*Lilly*) is a proprietary ANTIBIOTIC drug, available only on prescription, used primarily to treat infections in the urinary tract. Produced in the form of capsules, Cinobac is a preparation of cinoxacin. It is not recommended for children.

▲/✚ side-effects/warning: CINOXACIN.

cinoxacin is an ANTIBIOTIC of the quinolone family used primarily to treat infections in the urinary tract. Administration is oral in the form of capsules.

▲ side-effects: there may be nausea and vomiting, with

gastrointestinal disturbances and weight loss, diarrhoea and cramps. Some patients experience sensitivity reactions, including a rash, dizziness, a headache and tinnitus.

✚ warning: cinoxacin should be administered with caution to patients with even slightly impaired kidney function. It is not recommended for children.
Related article: CINOBAC.

Claforan (*Roussel*) is a proprietary ANTIBIOTIC preparation, available only on prescription, used to treat many forms of infection, including meningitis. Produced in vials as a powder for reconstitution as a medium for injection, Claforan is a preparation of the CEPHALOSPORIN cefotaxime.
▲/✚ side-effects/warning: *see* CEFOTAXIME.

clavulanic acid is a weakly antibiotic substance which has the effect of inhibiting bacterial resistance in bacteria that have become resistant to some penicillin-type antibiotics, notably amoxycillin and ticarcillin. It is a potent inhibitor of bacterial penicillinase enzymes that can inactivate many antibiotics of the penicillin family. It is therefore used in combination with amoxycillin or ticarcillin to treat infective conditions in which the penicillin alone might be unsuccessful, and has the additional effect of extending the activity of the antibiotic.
Related article: AUGMENTIN; TIMENTIN.

clindamycin is a broad-spectrum ANTIBIOTIC used to treat infections of bones and joints, and to assist in the treatment of peritonitis (inflammation of the peritoneal lining of the abdominal cavity). It is notably active against many anaerobic bacteria. Administration is oral in the form of capsules or a dilute suspension, or by injection.
▲ side-effects: if diarrhoea or other symptoms of colitis appear during treatment, administration must be halted at once (*see below*). There may also be nausea and vomiting.

C

✚ warning: clindamycin should not be administered to patients suffering from diarrhoea; and if diarrhoea or other symptoms of colitis appear during treatment, administration must be halted at once. This is because clindamycin greatly alters the normal balance of bacteria in the gut and in a few cases this allows a superinfection by an anaerobe, *Clostridium difficile*, which causes a form of colitis, resulting in potentially severe symptoms. It should be administered with caution to those with impaired liver or kidney function.
Related article: DALACIN C.

Clinicide (*De Witt*) is a proprietary non-prescription preparation used to treat scalp and pubic infestations of lice (pediculosis). Produced in the form of a lotion, Clinicide's active constituent is CARBARYL.

clioquinol is an ANTISEPTIC compound that contains iodine and is effective against infections by amoebae and some other micro-organisms. Its primary use is to treat infections of the skin and the outer ear. Administration is topical (in the form of drops, creams, ointments and anal suppositories). Systemic use of the drug has been associated with serious toxicity of the optic nerve, causing blindness.
▲ side-effects: some patients experience sensitivity reactions.
✚ warning: prolonged or excessive use encourages the onset of fungal infection. The drug stains skin and fabric.
Related article: LOCORTEN-VIOFORM.

clofazimine is a drug used as part of the treatment of the major form of leprosy, in combination with dapsone and rifampicin. That the treatment requires no fewer than three drugs is due to the increasing resistance shown by the leprotic bacterium. Administration is oral in the form of capsules.
▲ side-effects: there may be nausea and giddiness, diarrhoea and headache. High dosage may cause the

skin and the urine to take on a reddish tinge and a blue-black discoloration of skin lesions.

✚ warning: clofamizine should be administered with caution to patients with impaired kidney or liver function. Regular tests on both functions are essential.

clomocycline sodium is a broad-spectrum ANTIBIOTIC, one of the TETRACYCLINES, used to treat many forms of infection caused by several types of micro-organism. It is used particularly to treat infections of the urinary tract, the respiratory tract, and genital organs, and acne. Administration is oral in the form of capsules.

▲ side-effects: there may be nausea and vomiting, with diarrhoea. Occasionally there is sensitivity to light or other sensitivity reaction.

✚ warning: clomocycline sodium should not be administered to patients who are aged under 12 years, who are pregnant, or with impaired kidney function; it should be administered with caution to those who are lactating.

Related article: MEGACLOR.

clotrimazole is an ANTIFUNGAL drug used in topical application to treat fungal infection on the skin and mucous membranes (especially the vagina, the outer ear and the toes). Administration is in the form of a water-miscible cream, a dusting-powder, a spray, vaginal inserts (pessaries), and a lotion (solution).

▲ side-effects: rarely, there is a burning sensation or irritation; a very few patients experience sensitivity reactions.

Related article: CANESTEN.

cloxacillin is an ANTIBIOTIC of the penicillin family, used primarily to treat forms of infection which other penicillins are incapable of countering, due to the production of the enzyme penicillinase by the bacteria concerned. However, cloxacillin is not inactivated by the penicillinase enzymes produced, for example, by certain Staphylococci. It is therefore classed as a penicillinase-resistant penicillin. Administration is oral in the form of capsules and a dilute syrup, and by injection.

▲ side-effects: there may be sensitivity reactions ranging from a minor rash to urticaria and joint pains, fever or anaphylactic shock.

✚ warning: cloxacillin should not be administered to patients who are known to be allergic to penicillins; it should be administered with caution to those with impaired kidney function.

Related articles: AMPICLOX; ORBENIN.

colistin is a comparatively toxic ANTIBIOTIC of the polymyxin type that is used in topical application (in the form of colistin sulphate) to treat infections of the skin, and particularly the ears. However, in certain conditions and under strict supervision, the drug may be administered orally (primarily to sterilize the bowel, it is not absorbed) or by injection (primarily to treat urinary infection).

▲ side-effects: there may be breathlessness, vertigo, numbness round the mouth, and muscular weakness. Treatment by injection may cause symptoms of nerve or kidney disease.

✚ warning: colistin should not be administered to patients who suffer from the neuromuscular disease myasthenia gravis; it should be administered with caution to those who suffer from impaired kidney function. Dosage by injection is in millions of units.

Related article: COLOMYCIN.

Colomycin (*Pharmax*) is a proprietary form of the ANTIBIOTIC colistin sulphate, available only on prescription. In powder form, it is used mainly in topical application to treat skin infections, burns and wounds. It is also produced in the form of tablets, and as a syrup for dilution (the potency of the syrup once diluted is retained for 14 days), and (in the form of colistin sulphomethate sodium) as a powder for reconstitution as a medium for injection.

▲/✚ side-effects/warning: *see* COLISTIN.

Combantrin (*Pfizer*) is a proprietary broad-spectrum ANTHELMINTIC preparation, available only on prescription, used to treat infestations by roundworm, threadworm, hookworm and whipworm. Produced in the form of tablets, Combantrin is a preparation of pyrantel embonate. It is not recommended for children aged under 6 months.

▲✚ side-effects/warning: *see* PYRANTEL.

Comox (*Norton*) is a proprietary broad-spectrum ANTIBIOTIC drug, available only on prescription, used to treat infections of the urinary tract, the sinuses or the middle ear, and diseases such as typhoid fever or exacerbations of chronic bronchitis. Produced in the form of tablets (in two strengths, the stronger under the name Comox Forte), as soluble (dispersible) tablets, and as a suspension for children, Comox is a compound of the SULPHONAMIDE sulphamethoxazole and trimethoprim − a compound itself known as CO-TRIMOXAZOLE.

▲✚ side-effects/warning: *see* SULPHAMETHOXAZOLE; TRIMETHOPRIM.

Comprecin (*P-D*) is a proprietary ANTIBIOTIC preparation available only on prescription, used to treat gonorrhoea and bacterial dysentery and infections of the urinary tract and skin. Produced in the form of tablets, Comprecin is a preparation of the quinolone antibiotic enoxacin. It is not recommended for use in children.

▲✚ side-effects/warning: *see* ENOXACIN.

Conotrane (*Boehringer Ingelheim*) is a proprietary non-prescription ANTISEPTIC preparation, used to treat rash and sores and for skin protection. Produced in the form of cream, Conotrane is a preparation of BENZALKONIUM CHLORIDE and dimethicone '350' and a fragrance.

Corsodyl (*ICI*) is a proprietary non-prescription ANTISEPTIC preparation, used in topical application to treat inflammations and infections of the mouth. Produced in the form of a gel and as a mouth-wash, Corsodyl is a preparation of CHLORHEXIDINE gluconate.

corticosteroids are steroid hormones secreted by the cortex (outer part) of the adrenal glands, or synthetic substances that closely resemble them. There are two main types: glucocorticoids and mineralocorticoids. The latter assist in maintaining the salt and water balance of the body. The glucocorticoids are potent anti-inflammatory agents, frequently used to treat inflammatory and/or allergic reactions of the skin. Such reactions are sometimes complicated by a co-existing infection, and so many drug companies produce compound preparations containing both an antibiotic (or an antifungal) and an anti-inflammatory corticosteroid. Caution must be exercised in their use because the corticosteroid diminishes the patient's immune response to the infective agent, placing even greater reliance on the antibiotic or antifungal agent. Absorption of a high dose of corticosteroid over a period of time may also cause other undesirable systemic side-effects, such as peptic ulceration, brittle bones, muscle disorders, stunting of growth in children and accumulation of tissue fluids.

co-trimoxazole is the name for an ANTIBIOTIC combination of the SULPHONAMIDE sulphamethoxazole and the similar but not related trimethoprim (a folic acid inhibitor). At one time it was thought that each agent enhanced the action of the other, giving a combined effect greater than the sum of the two. While there is in fact little evidence to support this, the combination remains a very useful antibiotic preparation. It is used to treat and to prevent the spread of infections of the urinary tract, the nasal passages and upper respiratory tract, and the bones and joints, and such diseases as typhoid fever or gonorrhoea (particularly in patients allergic to penicillin); it is the active constituent of many proprietary antibiotic preparations. Administration is oral in the form of tablets or suspension, or by injection or infusion. Side-effects are largely due to the sulphonamide.
▲ side-effects: there may be nausea and vomiting; rashes are not uncommon. Blood disorders may occur.
✚ warning: co-trimoxazole should not be administered to patients who are pregnant or with blood disorders,

jaundice, or impaired liver or kidney function. It should be administered with caution to infants under 6 weeks and those who are elderly or lactating. Adequate fluid intake must be maintained. Prolonged treatment requires regular blood counts.

Related articles: BACTRIM; CHEMOTRIM; COMOX; FECTRIM; LARATRIM; SEPTRIN.

crystal violet is another name for gentian violet.
see GENTIAN VIOLET.

Crystapen (*Glaxo*) is a proprietary ANTIBIOTIC, available only on prescription, used to treat infections of the skin, of the middle ear, and of the respiratory tract (such as tonsillitis), and certain severe systemic infections (such as meningitis). Produced as a powder for reconstitution in any of three forms suited to specific sites of injection, Crystapen is a preparation of benzylpenicillin sodium.
▲/✚ side-effects/warning: *see* BENZYLPENICILLIN.

Crystapen V (*Glaxo*) is a proprietary ANTIBIOTIC, available only on prescription, used to treat many forms of infection, and to prevent rheumatic fever. Produced in the form of a syrup (in two strengths) for dilution (the potency of the syrup once diluted is retained for 7 days), Crystapen V is a preparation of phenoxymethylpenicillin.
▲/✚ side-effects/warning: *see* PHENOXYMETHYLPENICILLIN.

cycloserine is an ANTIBIOTIC drug used specifically in the treatment of tuberculosis that proves to be resistant to the powerful drugs ordinarily used first, or in cases where those drugs are not tolerated. Administration is oral in the form of capsules.
▲ side-effects: there may be headache, dizziness, and drowsiness; possible sensitivity reactions include a rash or, rarely, convulsions.
✚ warning: cycloserine should not be administered to patients with epilepsy, alcoholism, depressive illness, anxiety or psychosis; it should be administered with caution to those with impaired kidney function.

Daktacort (*Janssen*) is a proprietary cream for topical application, available only on prescription, that contains the CORTICOSTEROID hydrocortisone and the ANTIFUNGAL agent miconazole nitrate in a water-miscible base. It is used to treat skin inflammation in which fungal infection is also present.
▲/✚ side-effects/warning: *see* MICONAZOLE.

Daktarin (*Janssen*) is a proprietary ANTIFUNGAL drug, available only on prescription, used to treat both systemic and skin-surface fungal infections. Produced in the form of tablets and as a solution for infusion (after dilution), Daktarin is a preparation of the imidazole antifungal MICONAZOLE. Three other versions are available without prescription, in the form of a sugar-free gel for oral treatment, and a water-miscible cream and a spray powder in an aerosol for topical application.
▲/✚ side-effects/warning: *see* MICONAZOLE.

Dalacin C (*Upjohn*) is a proprietary ANTIBIOTIC, available only on prescription, used to treat staphylococcal infections of bones and joints, and peritonitis (inflammation of the peritoneal lining of the abdominal cavity). Produced in the form of capsules (in two strengths), as a paediatric suspension for dilution (the potency of the suspension once diluted is retained for 14 days), and in ampoules for injection, Dalacin C is a preparation of clindamycin. Side-effects are potentially severe.
▲/✚ side-effects/warning: *see* CLINDAMYCIN.

Dalacin T (*Upjohn*) is a proprietary ANTIBIOTIC available only on prescription, used to treat acne. Produced in the form of a solution for topical application, it is a preparation of the antibiotic clindamycin phosphate; not recommended for children. The serious colitis, which affects a small percentage of patients who take clindamycin orally, is not a problem with the topical use of this product.
▲/✚ side-effects/warning: *see* CLINDAMYCIN.

dapsone is an ANTIBIOTIC compound used specifically to treat leprosy (in both lepromatous and tuberculoid forms); it is also sometimes used to treat severe forms of dermatitis or, in combination with the enzyme-inhibitor pyrimethamine (under the trade name Maloprim), to prevent tropical travellers from contracting malaria. Administration is oral in the form of tablets, or by injection.

✚ warning: dapsone should be administered with caution to patients with anaemia, porphyria, glucose-6-phosphenate dehydrogenase deficiency, heart or lung disease or who are pregnant or lactating.

▲ side-effects: side-effects are rare at low doses (as for leprosy), but with higher dosage there may be nausea, vomiting and headache, insomnia and increased heart rate, severe weight loss, anaemia, hepatitis, neuropathy or agranulocytosis .
Related article: MALOPRIM.

Daraprim (*Wellcome*) is a proprietary non-prescription ANTIMALARIAL drug used in combination with other antimalarials to prevent tropical travellers from contracting malaria. It is not recommended as the sole agent of prevention. It works by interfering with the cellular composition of the parasitic organism that causes malaria, but treatment must be continued for 4 weeks after leaving the area of exposure. A preparation of pyrimethamine, Daraprim is not recommended for children aged under 5 years.

▲/✚ side-effects/warning: *see* PYRIMETHAMINE.

demeclocycline hydrochloride is a broad-spectrum ANTIBIOTIC, one of the TETRACYCLINES, used to treat infections of many kinds. Administration is oral in the form of tablets and capsules.

✚ warning: demeclocycline hydrochloride should not be administered to patients with kidney failure, who are pregnant, or who are aged under 12 years. It should be administered with caution to those who are lactating, or with impaired liver function.

▲ side-effects: there may be nausea and vomiting, with diarrhoea. Some patients experience a sensitivity to light. Rarely, there are allergic reactions.
Related articles: DETECLO; LEDERMYCIN; TETRACYCLINE.

Dequadin (*Farley*) is the name of a proprietary non-prescription lozenge containing the mild ANTIFUNGAL agent dequalinium chloride, to be sucked slowly until it dissolves, so treating oral infections.

dequalinium chloride is a mild ANTIFUNGAL agent that also has some antibacterial properties. It is used primarily to treat fungal infections of the mouth and throat (such as thrush). Administration is oral in the form of lozenges, or topical in the form of a paint.
Related article: DEQUADIN.

Derbac-C (*International Labs*) is a proprietary non-prescription drug used to treat infestations of the scalp and pubic hair by lice (pediculosis). Produced in the form of a shampoo, Derbac-C (also called Derbac Shampoo) is a preparation of the pediculicide carbaryl.
▲/✚ side-effects/warning: *see* CARBARYL.

Derbac-M (*International Labs*) is a proprietary non-prescription drug used to treat infestations of the scalp and pubic hair by lice (pediculosis), or of the skin by the itch-mite (scabies). Produced in the form of a lotion, Derbac-M is a preparation of the insecticide malathion.
✚ warning: *see* MALATHION.

Derbac Shampoo is another name for Derbac-C.
see DERBAC-C.

Dermonistat (*Ortho-Cilag*) is a proprietary non-prescription ANTIFUNGAL cream used to treat infections of the skin and the nails. Topical treatment must be continued for 10 days after the infective lesions have disappeared. Dermonistat is a preparation of the imidazole antifungal, miconazole nitrate.
▲/✚ side-effects/warning: *see* MICONAZOLE.

D

Dermovate-NN (*Glaxo*) is a combined ANTIBIOTIC, ANTIFUNGAL and CORTICOSTEROID preparation for topical application, available only on prescription, used (in the short term only) to treat severe exacerbations in serious inflammatory skin disorders such as discoid lupus erythematosus. Produced in the form of a cream, and as an ointment in an anhydrous base for dilution with white soft paraffin (the potency of the ointment once diluted is retained for 14 days), Dermovate-NN is in both forms a preparation of the steroid clobetasol propionate with the broad-spectrum antibiotic neomycin sulphate and the antifungal agent nystatin.

▲/✚ side-effects/warning: *see* NEOMYCIN; NYSTATIN.

Deteclo (*Lederle*) is a proprietary compound ANTIBIOTIC preparation, available only on prescription, used to treat many kinds of infection, but especially those of the respiratory tract, the ear, nose and throat, the gastrointestinal tract and the genito-urinary tract, and the soft tissues. Deteclo consists of a combination of TETRACYCLINES − chlortetracycline hydrochloride, tetracycline hydrochloride and demeclocycline hydrochloride − and is produced in the form of tablets. It should not be used for children under the age of 12 years, and should not be given to pregnant women or patients with kidney disease.

▲/✚ side-effects/warning: *see* CHLORTETRACYCLINE; DEMECLOCYCLINE HYDROCHLORIDE; TETRACYCLINE.

Dettol (*Reckitt & Colman*) is a well-known proprietary non-prescription ANTISEPTIC lotion, used for ordinary disinfectant purposes or in treating abrasions and minor wounds. But it is also used in obstetrics for the antisepsis of hands, gloves and forceps, and as a vaginal lubricant during labour. It is a preparation of CHLOROXYLENOL (in mild solution).

diethylcarbamazine citrate is an ANTHELMINTIC, specifically an antifilarial agent used to treat infestation by filarial worm parasites (such as those that cause elephantiasis, lymphangitis, loiasis and onchocerciasis). Side-effects are inevitable but are generally treated in turn with other drugs; close monitoring is essential throughout treatment, particularly at first. Several courses of treatment may be necessary. Administration is oral in the form of tablets.

▲ side-effects: there may be nausea and vomiting, with headache. Skin and eye inflammations may be aggravated.

✚ warning: the destruction of the worm-parasites causes the release of antigens and the corresponding allergic response which manifest themselves in skin irritation and inflammation, and visual disturbances because the eyes are also affected. Antihistamines and corticosteroids may be prescribed to deal with these. *Related article:* BANOCIDE.

Diflucan (*Pfizer*) is a proprietary ANTIFUNGAL drug available only on prescription, used to treat candidiasis (thrush) of the vagina or mouth. Produced in the form of capsules in two strengths, it is an orally active preparation of fluconazole.

▲/✚ side-effects/warning: *see* FLUCONAZOLE.

diloxanide furoate is an AMOEBICIDAL drug used to treat chronic infection of the intestine by amoebae, causing amoebic dysentery. Administration is oral in the form of tablets; the drug is given in combination with the antibiotic metronidazole in acute cases.

▲ side-effects: there is usually flatulence; there may also be vomiting, itching (pruritus) and/or urticaria.

✚ warning: treatment with diloxanide furoate alone usually lasts 10 days; with metronidazole 15 days. *Related article:* FURAMIDE.

diphtheria antitoxin is a preparation of antibodies to the toxin produced by the diphtheria bacteria, *Corynebacterium diphtheriae*, as this toxin is the major factor in the lethal complications of diphtheria infections. The antibodies are prepared in horses, and once used in patients carry the risk of sensitization of the patient to horse proteins. The antitoxin absorbed onto a carrier, usually aluminium hydroxide, causes active immunity in the patient. It is the mainstay of treatment of suspected and proven cases of diphtheria. Prior tests for sensitization should be carried out.

diphtheria vaccine is a VACCINE preparation of an inactivated, yet still antigenic, toxin (or toxoid) of the diphtheria bacteria, *Corynebacterium diphtheriae*. Available only on prescription, the vaccine is produced in ampoules for injection. However, far more commonly, it is administered as one constituent in a triple vaccine (additionally against whooping cough − known as pertussis − and tetanus, often called the DPT vaccine) or, when patients do not want vaccination against whooping cough, in a double vaccine (with TETANUS VACCINE). Reinforcing doses of diphtheria vaccine are required.

diphtheria-pertussis-tetanus (DPT) vaccine is a combination of VACCINES against diphtheria, whooping cough and tetanus used for the routine immunization of infants at the ages of 3 months, 4+ months and 6 months. Repeat vaccination with this triple vaccine is not usual, although the booster vaccinations of the diphtheria and tetanus vaccines are relatively common.
see DIPHTHERIA VACCINE; PERTUSSIS VACCINE; TETANUS VACCINE.

diphtheria-tetanus vaccine is a combination of VACCINES against diphtheria and tetanus used for the routine immunization of infants at the ages of 3 months, 4+ months and 6 months in children whose parents do not wish them to have the triple vaccine that additionally contains pertussis (whooping cough) vaccine. This double vaccine is also used as a booster shot for children at the age of school entry.

Disadine DP (*Stuart*) is a proprietary non-prescription form of the compound DISINFECTANT povidone-iodine, prepared as a powder within an aerosol. For topical application, it is used to treat or prevent infection of the skin following injury or surgery, or to cleanse bedsores.

*disinfectants are agents that destroy micro-organisms, or inhibit their activity to a level such that they are less or no longer harmful to health. The term is applied to agents used on inanimate objects as well as to those used to treat the skin and living tissue, and in the latter case is often used synonymously with ANTISEPTIC.

Dispray 1 Quick Prep (*Stuart*) is a proprietary non-prescription DISINFECTANT used primarily to cleanse the skin prior to surgery or injection. Produced in an aerosol for immediate topical application, it is a solution of CHLORHEXIDINE GLUCONATE.

Distaclor (*Dista*) is a proprietary broad-spectrum ANTIBIOTIC, available only on prescription, used to treat a wide range of bacterial infections, particularly of the skin and soft tissues, urinary tract, upper respiratory tract, and middle ear. Produced in the form of capsules and as a suspension (in two strengths) for dilution (the potency of the suspension once diluted is retained for 14 days), Distaclor is a preparation of the CEPHALOSPORIN CEFACLOR.
▲/✚ side-effects/warning: *see* CEFACLOR.

Distaquaine V-K (*Dista*) is a proprietary preparation of the penicillin-type ANTIBIOTIC phenoxymethylpenicillin, used mainly to treat infections of the throat, middle ear and some skin conditions. Available only on prescription, it is produced in the form of tablets (in two strengths) or as an elixir (in three strengths) for dilution (the potency of the elixir once diluted is retained for 7 days).
▲/✚ side-effects/warning: *see* PHENOXYMETHYLPENICILLIN.

Doxatet (*Cox Pharmaceuticals*) is a proprietary broad-spectrum ANTIBIOTIC, available only on prescription, used to treat infections of many kinds. Produced in the form of tablets, Doxatet is a preparation of the TETRACYCLINE doxycycline hydrochloride. It is not recommended for children.

▲/✚ side-effects/warning: *see* DOXYCYCLINE.

doxycycline is a broad-spectrum ANTIBIOTIC, one of the TETRACYCLINES, used to treat infections of many kinds, notably chlamydial infections (including urethritis and psittacosis), myocaplasmal (pneumonia) infections and exacerbations of chronic bronchitis due to *Haemophilus influenzae*. Administration is oral in the form of tablets and capsules, soluble (dispersible) tablets for solution, and as a dilute syrup. Unlike most tetracyclines it is relatively non-toxic to the kidney.

▲ side-effects: there may be nausea and vomiting, with diarrhoea. Some patients experience a sensitivity to light. Rarely, there are allergic reactions.

✚ warning: doxycycline should be administered with care to patients who are pregnant, or who are aged under 12 years. It should be administered with care to patients who are lactating.

Related articles: DOXATET; DOXYLAR; NORDOX; VIBRAMYCIN.

Doxylar (*Lagap*) is a proprietary broad-spectrum ANTIBIOTIC, available only on prescription, used to treat infections of many kinds. Produced in the form of capsules, Doxylar is a preparation of the TETRACYCLINE doxycycline hydrochloride.

▲/✚ side-effects/warning: *see* DOXYCYCLINE.

Drapolene (*Wellcome*) is a proprietary non-prescription ANTISEPTIC cream used primarily to treat nappy rash, although it can also be used to dress abrasions and minor wounds. It contains the antiseptics BENZALKONIUM CHLORIDE and CETRIMIDE in very dilute solution.

Econacort (*Squibb*) is a proprietary preparation that combines the CORTICOSTEROID hydrocortisone with the ANTIFUNGAL econazole nitrate. Available only on prescription and produced in the form of a cream for topical application, Econacort is used to treat inflammation in which fungal infection is also diagnosed. The cream, applied sparingly, should be massaged into the skin; prolonged use should be avoided.

▲/✚ side-effects/warning: *see* ECONAZOLE NITRATE.

econazole nitrate is a broad-spectrum ANTIFUNGAL agent, one of the IMIDAZOLES, used particularly in topical applications to treat fungal infections of the skin or mucous membranes, such as vaginal candidiasis. Administration is in the form of creams or ointments, as vaginal inserts (pessaries or tampons), or as lotions, sprays or dusting-powders.

▲ side-effects: there may be local skin irritation, even to the extent of a burning sensation and redness.
Related articles: ECOSTATIN; GYNO-PEVARYL; PEVARYL.

Econocil VK (*DDSA Pharmaceuticals*) is a proprietary preparation of the penicillin-type ANTIBIOTIC phenoxymethylpenicillin. It is effective orally, and used mainly to treat infections of the middle ear and throat, and some skin conditions. Available only on prescription, it is produced in the form of capsules and tablets (in two strengths).

▲/✚ side-effects/warning: *see* PHENOXYMETHYLPENICILLIN.

Economycin (*DDSA Pharmaceuticals*) is a proprietary ANTIBIOTIC, available only on prescription, used to treat many kinds of infection, but especially those of the respiratory tract, ear, nose and throat, gastrointestinal tract, urinary tract, and soft tissues. Produced in the form of capsules and tablets, Economycin is a preparation of the TETRACYCLINE tetracycline hydrochloride.

▲/✚ side-effects/warning: *see* TETRACYCLINE.

Ecostatin (*Squibb*) is a proprietary non-prescription

ANTIFUNGAL preparation of econazole nitrate, used primarily to treat yeast infections of the skin and mucous membranes, especially in the urogenital areas. It is produced (in solution) in the form of a water-miscible cream, as a lotion, as a spray for topical application, as a dusting-powder, as a talc-based powder in a spray container, and as vaginal inserts (pessaries). Treatment should continue for at least a fortnight after lesions have disappeared.

▲ side-effects: see ECONAZOLE NITRATE.

Eludril (*Concept*) is a proprietary non-prescription mouth-wash that has ANTIBACTERIAL and ANTIFUNGAL properties and inhibits the formation of plaque on the teeth. It is also used in the treatment of gum disease and mouth ulcers. Containing the ANTISEPTIC chlorhexidine gluconate and chlorbutol, Eludril is not recommended for children aged under 6 years. An aerosol spray version is also available.

▲/✚ side-effects/warning: *see* CHLORHEXIDINE.

enoxacin is an antibiotic drug of the quinolone family, used to treat infections of the urinary tract and skin, gonorrhoea and bacterial dysentery. Administration is oral in the form of tablets.

▲ side-effects: there may be nausea and vomiting, with gastro-intestinal disturbances and weight loss, diarrhoea and cramps. Some patients experience sensitivity reactions including a rash, dizziness, headache and ringing in the ears.

✚ warning: enoxacin should be administered with caution to patients with even slightly impaired kidney function.

Enteromide (*Consolidated*) is a proprietary ANTIBIOTIC drug, available only on prescription, formerly used to treat inflammation and infection of the intestines, to relieve food poisoning, or to reduce bacterial levels in the intestines before surgery or examination, but now used less commonly. Produced in the form of tablets, Enteromide is a preparation of the poorly absorbed SULPHONAMIDE drug calcium sulphaloxate.

▲/✚ side-effects/warning: *see* CALCIUM SULPHALOXATE.

Eradacin (*Sterling Research*) is a proprietary preparation of the ANTIBIOTIC drug acrosoxacin, one of the quinolones, available only on prescription, used to treat the sexually transmitted disease gonorrhoea in patients who are allergic to penicillin, or whose strain of gonorrhoea is resistant to penicillin-type antibiotics. Produced in the form of capsules, Eradacin is not recommended for children.

▲/✚ side-effects/warning: *see* ACROSOXACIN.

Ervevax (*Smith, Kline & French*) is a proprietary VACCINE against German measles (rubella) in the form of a solution containing live but attenuated viruses of the Wistar RA27/3 strain. Available only on prescription, it is administered in the form of injection.

Erycen (*Berk*) is a proprietary ANTIBIOTIC, available only on prescription, used to treat many forms of infection (particularly pneumonia and legionnaires' disease) and to prevent others (particularly sinusitis, diphtheria and whooping cough), and as an alternative to penicillin-type antibiotics in patients who are allergic or whose infections are resistant. Produced in the form of tablets (in two strengths) and a suspension, Erycen is a preparation of the macrolide erythromycin. It is not recommended for children.

▲/✚ side-effects/warning: *see* ERYTHROMYCIN.

Erymax (*Parke-Davis*) is a proprietary ANTIBIOTIC, available only on prescription, used to treat many forms of infection (particularly pneumonia and legionnaires' disease) and to prevent others (particularly sinusitis, diphtheria and whooping cough), and as an alternative to penicillin-type antibiotics in patients who are allergic or whose infections are resistant. Produced in the form of capsules, Erymax is a preparation of the macrolide erythromycin. Also available is Erymax sprinkle, a preparation produced in the form of capsules whose contents may be sprinkled on soft food for use in children.

▲/✚ side-effects/warning: *see* ERYTHROMYCIN.

E

Erythrocin (*Abbott*) is a proprietary ANTIBIOTIC, available only on prescription, used to treat many forms of infection (particularly pneumonia and legionnaires' disease) and to prevent others (particularly sinusitis, diphtheria and whooping cough), and as an alternative to penicillin-type antibiotics in patients who are allergic or whose infections are resistant. Produced in the form of tablets (in two strengths), and as a powder for reconstitution as a medium for injection, Erythrocin is a preparation of salts of the macrolide erythromycin. The tablets are not recommended for children.

▲/✚ side-effects/warning: *see* ERYTHROMYCIN.

Erythrolar (*Lagap*) is a proprietary ANTIBIOTIC, available only on prescription, used to treat many forms of infection (particularly pneumonia and legionnaires' disease) and to prevent others (particularly sinusitis, diphtheria and whooping cough) and as an alternative to penicillin-type antibiotics in patients who are allergic or whose infections are resistant. Produced in the form of tablets (in two strengths), and as a suspension for dilution (the potency of the suspension once diluted is retained for 5 days), Erythrolar is a preparation of salts of the macrolide erythromycin.

▲/✚ side-effects/warning: *see* ERYTHROMYCIN.

Erythromid (*Abbott*) is a proprietary ANTIBIOTIC, available only on prescription, used to treat many forms of infection (particularly pneumonia and legionnaires' disease) and to prevent others (particularly sinusitis, diphtheria and whooping cough), and as an alternative to penicillin-type antibiotics in patients who are allergic or whose infections are resistant. Produced in the form of tablets (in two strengths, the stronger under the name Erythromid DS), Erythromid is a preparation of the macrolide erythromycin. It is not recommended for children.

▲/✚ side-effects/warning: *see* ERYTHROMYCIN.

erythromycin is a macrolide ANTIBIOTIC with a similar spectrum of action to penicillin, but a different mechanism of action: it inhibits microbial protein synthesis at the ribosome level. It is effective against many gram-positive bacteria including streptococci (soft tissue and respiratory tract infections), mycoplasma (pneumonia), legionella (legionnaire's disease) and chlamydia (urethritis). It is also used as prophylaxis (preventative therapy) for diphtheria and whooping cough. Erythromycin's principal use is as an alternative to penicillin in individuals who are allergic to penicillin. Bacterial resistance is unfortunately not uncommon. Administration is oral in the form of tablets, as capsules, or as a dilute suspension (mixture), or by injection. Tablets have to be enteric- or film-coated because the drug is inactivated by gastric secretions.

▲ side-effects: large doses may cause nausea and vomiting, and possibly diarrhoea.

✚ warning: one salt of erythromycin (the estolate), a constituent in a proprietary suspension, should not be administered to patients with liver disease; all forms of the drug should be administered with caution to those with impaired liver function.

Related articles: ARPIMYCIN; ERYCEN; ERYMAX; ERYTHROCIN; ERYTHROLAR; ERYTHROMID; ERYTHROPED; ILOSONE; ILOTYCIN; RETCIN.

Erythroped (*Abbott*) is a proprietary ANTIBIOTIC, available only on prescription, used to treat many forms of infection (particularly pneumonia and legionnaires' disease) and to prevent others (particularly sinusitis, diphtheria and whooping cough), and as an alternative to penicillin-type antibiotics in patients who are allergic or whose infections are resistant. Produced in the form of a suspension (in three strengths) for dilution (the potency of the suspension once diluted is retained for 5 days), as sugar-free granules in sachets for solution, and as tablets (under the name Erythroped A), Erythroped is a preparation of salts of the macrolide erythromycin.

▲/✚ side-effects/warning: *see* ERYTHROMYCIN.

Esoderm (*Napp*) is a proprietary non-prescription

E

preparation of the drug lindane, used to treat parasitic
infestation by lice (pediculosis) or by itch-mites (scabies)
on the skin surface, particularly under the hair. However,
strains of head-lice resistant to lindane have recently
emerged, and the drug is not now recommended for use
on the scalp. It is produced in the form of a (flammable)
alcohol-based lotion, and as a cream shampoo.
▲/✚ side-effects/warning: *see* LINDANE.

ethambutol hydrochloride is an ANTIBIOTIC that is one of
the major forms of treatment for tuberculosis. Even so, it
is used generally in combination (to cover resistance and
for maximum effect) with other antitubercular drugs such
as isoniazid or rifampicin. Treatment lasts for between 6
and 9 months depending on severity and on the specific
drug combination, but the use of ethambutol tends to
imply the shorter duration. The drug is also used to
prevent the contraction of tuberculosis by relatives.
Administration is oral in the form of tablets or as a
powder.

▲ side-effects: side-effects are rare, and are mostly in the
form of visual disturbances (such as loss of acuity or
colour-blindness) which should prove temporary if
treatment is withdrawn. A regular ophthalmic check is
advised during treatment.

✚ warning: ethambutol hydrochloride should not be
administered to children aged under 6 years, to
patients who are elderly, or to those who suffer from
nervous disorders of the eyes. It should be avoided in
patients with poor kidney function.

Related articles: MYAMBUTOL; MYNAH.

Exelderm (*ICI*) is a proprietary ANTIFUNGAL cream,
available only on prescription, used for topical application
to skin infections, such as athlete's foot or thrush. The
cream should be massaged into the skin; treatment
should continue for at least a fortnight after lesions have
disappeared. Exelderm is a preparation of the IMIDAZOLE
sulconazole nitrate.

▲/✚ side-effects/warning: *see* SULCONAZOLE NITRATE.

F

Fansidar (*Roche*) is a proprietary ANTIMALARIAL drug, available only on prescription, used — following a course of quinine — to treat patients who are seriously ill with malaria, particularly with strains resistant to the standard drug chloroquine. (A very few strains are resistant also to Fansidar.) It has been used prophylactically to try to prevent tropical travellers from contracting the disease, but is not now recommended for this purpose. Produced in the form of tablets, Fansidar is a compound of (the antimalarial) pyrimethamine together with the SULPHONAMIDE sulfadoxine. Dosage is critical, and must be carefully monitored.
▲/✚ side-effects/warning: *see* PYRIMETHAMINE.

Fasigyn (*Pfizer*) is a proprietary drug with ANTIBIOTIC and ANTIPROTOZOAL properties, available only on prescription, used to treat infections by anaerobic bacteria and protozoa, particularly in the gut, the vagina or on the gums, and to ensure asepsis during surgery. Produced in the form of tablets and as fluid in (two sizes of) flasks for intravenous infusion, Fasigyn is a preparation of the nitroimidazole drug tinidazole.
▲/✚ side-effects/warning: *see* TINIDAZOLE.

Fectrim (*DDSA Pharmaceuticals*) is a proprietary ANTIBIOTIC combination available only on prescription, used especially in infections of the urinary tract, infections of the respiratory tract, such as sinusitis and bronchitis, and infections of the bones and joints. Produced in the form of soluble (dispersible) tablets (in any of three strengths), Fectrim is a preparation of the compound drug co-trimoxazole, made up of the SULPHONAMIDE sulphamethoxazole together with the antibacterial agent TRIMETHOPRIM.
▲/✚ side-effects/warning: *see* CO-TRIMOXAZOLE.

Flagyl (*May & Baker*) is a proprietary form of the drug metronidazole, which has both ANTIPROTOZOAL and ANTIBIOTIC (specifically against anaerobic bacteria) properties. It is available only on prescription and is used

F

to treat anaerobic infections that may occur following colonic or gynaecological trauma or surgery. Brain abscess and Vincent's infections of the gums or throat are other bacterial infections it may also be used to treat. Flagyl's antiprotozoal activity is effective against the organisms that cause amoebic dysentery, giardiasis and trichomoniasis. It is produced in the form of capsules (in two strengths); in the form of a suspension for dilution it is called Flagyl S. Simultaneous treatment with anticoagulants or barbiturates should be avoided as should the consumption of alcohol.

▲/✚ side-effects/warning: *see* METRONIDAZOLE.

Flagyl Compak (*May & Baker*) is a proprietary combination of the ANTIPROTOZOAL drug, metronidazole and the ANTIFUNGAL nystatin. Available only on prescription, it is used to treat mixed infections of the vagina, including trichomoniasis and candidiasis.

▲/✚ side-effects/warning: *see* METRONIDAZOLE.

Flamazine (*Smith & Nephew*) is a proprietary ANTIBACTERIAL cream, available only on prescription, used to treat wounds, burns and ulcers, bedsores and skin-graft donor sites. It is a preparation of silver sulphadiazine in a water-soluble base.

▲/✚ side-effects/warning: *see* SILVER SULPHADIAZINE.

Floxapen (*Beecham*) is a proprietary ANTIBIOTIC, available only on prescription, used to treat bacterial infections of the skin and of the ear, nose and throat, and especially staphylococcal infections that prove to be resistant to penicillin. Produced in the form of capsules (in two strengths), syrup for dilution (in two strengths; the potency of the diluted syrup is retained for 14 days), and as a powder for reconstitution as injections, Floxapen's active constituent in each case is the penicillinase-resistant penicillin flucloxacillin, or one of its salts.

▲/✚ side-effects/warning: *see* FLUCLOXACILLIN.

Flu-Amp (*Generics*) is a proprietary compound ANTIBIOTIC available only on prescription used to treat bacterial infections particularly of the urinary tract, the middle ear and the upper respiratory tract. Produced in the form of capsules, Flu-Amp contains the penicillin ampicillin, together with the broad-spectrum penicillinase-resistant flucloxacillin (which can treat infections that prove to be resistant to penicillin).

▲/✚ side-effects/warning: *see* AMPICILLIN; FLUCLOXACILLIN.

flucloxacillin is an ANTIBIOTIC of the penicillin family. Similar to penicillin, it is active against many gram-positive bacteria, but its principal attribute is that it is generally resistant to the enzymes secreted by penicillin-resistant stapylococcus aureus, called penicillinases (which can inactivate many penicillins). It is used to treat bacterial infections of the skin and of the ear, nose and throat, and especially staphylococcal infections that prove to be resistant to penicillin. Administration is in the form of capsules, dilute syrup and injection.

▲ side-effects: there may be sensitivity reactions, including high temperature; in some patients there is diarrhoea.

✚ warning: flucloxacillin should not be administered to patients who have a history of allergy to antibiotic substances, or who suffer from impairment of kidney function.

Related articles: FLOXAPEN; LADROPEN; STAFOXIL; STAPHCIL.

fluconazole is an ANTIFUNGAL drug of the triazole family, used in the treatment of fungal infections of the mucous membranes of the vagina or mouth.

▲ side-effects: may cause nausea, abdominal discomfort and headaches.

✚ warning: it should not be administered to patients with kidney dysfunction or during pregnancy.

flucytosine is an ANTIFUNGAL drug used to treat systemic infections by yeasts – infections such as systemic candidiasis. Administration is oral or by intravenous infusion.

▲ side-effects: there may be diarrhoea, with nausea and vomiting; rashes may occur. White blood cell numbers may be lowered.

✚ warning: flucytosine should be administered only with caution to patients who suffer from impaired function of the kidneys or liver, or from blood disorders; or who are pregnant or lactating. During treatment there should be regular blood counts and liver-function tests. *Related article:* ALCOBON.

Fluvirin (*Servier*) is the name of a series of proprietary flu VACCINES, all comprising inactivated surface antigens of different strains of the influenza virus. None is recommended for children aged under 4 years.

▲ side-effects: rarely, there is local reaction together with headache and high temperature.

✚ warning: like any flu vaccine, Fluvirin cannot control epidemics and should be used only − in what seems to be the appropriate strain − on people who are at high risk: the elderly, patients with cardiovascular problems, and medical staff. Fluvirin should not be administered to patients who are allergic to egg or chicken protein (in which vaccine viruses are cultured), or who are pregnant.

FML-Neo (*Allergan*) is a proprietary form of ANTIBIOTIC eye-drops, available only on prescription, used in cases where the inflammation is not primarily caused by infection. The active constituents of FML-Neo are the CORTICOSTEROID fluorometholone and the aminoglycoside antibiotic neomycin.

▲/✚ side-effects/warning: *see* NEOMYCIN.

Fortum (*Glaxo*) is a proprietary broad-spectrum ANTIBIOTIC, available only on prescription, used to treat bacterial infections, particularly infections of the respiratory tract, the ear, nose or throat, the skin, bones and joints, and more serious infections such as septicaemia and meningitis. Produced in the form of powder for reconstitution as a medium for injection or infusion,

Fortum is a preparation of the CEPHALOSPORIN ceftazidime.
▲/✚ side-effects/warning: *see* CEFTAZIDIME.

framycetin is an aminoglycoside ANTIBIOTIC, largely
restricted to oral and topical usage due to its toxicity. It is
not absorbed from the gastrointestinal tract and therefore
when given orally the aim is to kill off sensitive bacteria
in the gut prior to intestinal surgery. As with all
aminoglycoside antibiotics, framycetin is active against
some gram-positive and many gram-negative bacteria.
Preparations of framycetin most commonly involve its
sulphate form.

▲ side-effects: hypersensitive reactions may occur; there
  may be temporary kidney malfunction.
✚ warning: oral administration may cause malabsorption
  of nutrients; application to large areas of the skin may
  damage the organs of the ears. Framycetin should not
  be administered to patients who are pregnant, or to
  those with myasthenia gravis.
  Related articles: FRAMYCORT; FRAMYGEN; SOFRAMYCIN.

Framycort (*Fisons*) is a proprietary compound, available
only on prescription, combining the aminoglycoside
ANTIBIOTIC framycetin sulphate with the fairly potent
CORTICOSTEROID hydrocortisone acetate. It is used in the
form of an ointment to treat skin infections,
particularly on the face or in the urogenital area; as
eye-drops to treat bacterial infections such as
conjunctivitis; and as ear-drops for the treatment of
bacterial infections of the outer ear.
▲/✚ side-effects/warning: *see* FRAMYCETIN.

Framygen (*Fisons*) is a proprietary ANTIBIOTIC, available
only on prescription, used in the form of eye ointment and
eye-drops to treat infections on and around the eyes; as
ear-drops to treat infections of the outer ear; and as a
cream to treat bacterial skin infections. In all versions, its
active constituent is the aminoglycoside framycetin
sulphate in very mild solution.
▲/✚ side-effects/warning: *see* FRAMYCETIN.

F

Fucibet (*Leo*) is a proprietary compound, available only on prescription, combining the potent CORTICOSTEROID betamethasone with the ANTIBIOTIC fusidic acid. It is used to treat eczema in which bacterial infection is deemed to be present, and is produced in the form of a cream.
▲/✚ side-effects/warning: *see* FUSIDIC ACID.

Fucidin (*Leo*) is a proprietary narrow-spectrum ANTIBIOTIC, available only on prescription, used mainly against staphylococcal infections − especially infections of the skin and bone, as well as abscesses − that prove to be resistant to penicillin. It is produced in many forms: as tablets, as a suspension, as powder for reconstitution as a medium for infusion, as a gel (with or without a special applicator), as a cream, and as an ointment, all for use as indicated by the location of the infection, and all containing as their active constituent either fusidic acid or one of its salts (particularly sodium fusidate).
▲/✚ side-effects/warning: *see* FUSIDIC ACID.

Fucidin H (*Leo*) is a proprietary compound, available only on prescription, combining the ANTIBIOTIC sodium fusidate with the CORTICOSTEROID hydrocortisone, and used to treat skin inflammation considered to involve bacterial infection. It is produced in the form of an ointment, a cream or a gel.
▲/✚ side-effects/warning: *see* FUSIDIC ACID.

Fucithalmic (*Leo*) is a proprietary ANTIBIOTIC available only on prescription, used in the form of a gel to treat staphyloccocal infections on and around the eyes. Its active constituent is the antibiotic fusidic acid.
▲/✚ side-effects/warning: *see* FUSIDIC ACID.

Fulcin (*ICI*) is a proprietary ANTIFUNGAL drug, available only on prescription, used to treat fungal infections of the scalp, skin and nails. Produced in the form of tablets (in two strengths) and as a suspension, Fulcin is a preparation of the drug griseofulvin. Treatment may be required to continue over several weeks.
▲/✚ side-effects/warning: *see* GRISEOFULVIN.

*fungicidal drugs act to destroy fungal infection, and are also known as an antimycotic or antifungal drugs.
see ANTIFUNGAL DRUGS.

Fungilin (*Squibb*) is a proprietary form of the ANTIFUNGAL drug amphotericin. Available only on prescription, Fungilin is produced in the form of tablets and as a suspension, as lozenges, as an ointment and as a cream, and used in the appropriate form to treat fungal infections, especially candidiasis (thrush) of the mouth, gastrointestinal tract, vagina and skin.
▲/✚ side-effects/warning: *see* AMPHOTERICIN.

Fungizone (*Squibb*) is a proprietary form of the ANTIFUNGAL drug amphotericin. Available only on prescription, Fungizone is produced in the form of powder for reconstitution as a medium for intravenous infusion, and used to treat systemic fungal infections.
▲/✚ side-effects/warning: *see* AMPHOTERICIN.

Furadantin (*Norwich Eaton*) is a proprietary ANTIBIOTIC drug, available only on prescription, used to treat infections of the urinary tract. It is produced in the form of tablets (in two strengths) and as a suspension, the active constituent of which is nitrofurantoin.
▲/✚ side-effects/warning: *see* NITROFURANTOIN.

Furamide (*Boots*) is a proprietary form of the AMOEBICIDAL drug diloxanide furoate, available only on prescription, used to treat chronic infection by the organism *Entamoeba histolytica* where cysts are discernible in the faeces. It is produced in the form of tablets.
▲/✚ side-effects/warning: *see* DILOXANIDE FUROATE.

fusidic acid and its salts are narrow-spectrum ANTIBIOTICS used to treat staphylococcal infections − particularly infections of the skin or of bone − that prove to be resistant to penicillin.
▲ side-effects: local hypersensitivity reactions may occur;

rarely, there may be gastric upset, jaundice, and a reversible change in liver function.

➕ warning: treatment by infusion may require periodic testing of the patient's liver function. Keep fusidic acid ointment, cream and gel away from the eyes.

Related articles: FUCIBET; FUCIDIN; FUCIDIN H.

Galenomycin (*Galen*) is a proprietary ANTIBIOTIC, available only on prescription, used to treat infections of the soft tissues and the respiratory tract. Produced in the form of tablets, Galenomycin is a preparation of the TETRACYCLINE oxytetracycline dihydrate. It is not recommended for children.

▲/✚ side-effects/warning: *see* OXYTETRACYCLINE.

G

Gamimune-N (*Cutter*) is a proprietary preparation of human normal immunoglobulin (HNIG) as a solution in maltose, used by intravenous infusion to confer immediate immunity to such diseases as hepatitis A virus, measles (rubeola) and at least to some degree rubella (German measles), particularly in patients who cannot tolerate the administration of live (though weakened) viruses in vaccination therapies. Gamimune-N is primarily used as replacement therapy in patients born with certain immunodeficient conditions. It is available only on prescription, in vials (in three strengths).

✚ warning: see HNIG.

Gammabulin (*Immuno*) is a proprietary preparation of human normal immunoglobulin (HNIG) as an aqueous solution, used by intramuscular injection to confer immediate immunity to such diseases as hepatitis A virus, measles (rubeola) and at least to some degree rubella (German measles), particularly in patients who cannot tolerate the administration of live (though weakened) viruses in vaccination therapies. It is available only prescription, in vials.

✚ warning: see HNIG.

Gantrisin (*Roche*) is a proprietary ANTIBACTERIAL drug, available only on prescription, used primarily to treat infections of the urinary tract, but also to relieve lesser infections of the skin and soft tissues and the respiratory tract, and to treat bacillary dysentery. Produced in the form of tablets and as a syrup, Gantrisin is a preparation of the SULPHONAMIDE sulphafurazole.

G

Garamycin (*Kirby-Warrick*) is a proprietary ANTIBIOTIC, available only on prescription, used primarily in the form of drops to treat bacterial infections of the ear or eye. Garamycin is a preparation of the aminoglycoside gentamicin.

▲/✚ side-effects/warning: *see* GENTAMICIN.

gentamicin is a broad-spectrum ANTIBIOTIC, the most widely used of the aminoglycoside family, with activity against gram-positive bacteria but used primarily against serious infections caused by gram-negative bacteria. It is not orally absorbed and is therefore given by injection or infusion for the treatment of, for example, septicaemia, meningitis and infections of the heart (usually in conjunction with penicillin), the kidney and the prostate gland. Because of its toxicity to the ear (ototoxicity), potentially resulting in deafness, and its toxicity to the kidney (nephrotoxicity), treatment should be limited in duration. It is also available in the form of drops, creams and ointments for topical application.

▲ side-effects: prolonged or high dosage may be damaging to the ear, causing deafness and balance disorders; treatment must be discontinued if this occurs; there may also be reversible kidney damage.

✚ warning: gentamicin should not be administered to patients who are pregnant or who suffer from myasthenia gravis. It should be administered with caution to those with Parkinsonism. As the drug is excreted by the kidney, great care must be taken in patients with impaired kidney function. In such cases, and/or where dosage is high or prolonged, regular checks on gentamicin concentrations in the blood must be carried out.

Related articles: CIDOMYCIN; GARAMYCIN; GENTICIN; GENTISONE HC; LUGACIN; MINIMS GENTAMICIN.

gentian violet, or crystal violet, is an ANTISEPTIC dye used to treat certain bacterial and fungal skin infections, or abrasions and minor wounds. Administration is mostly in the form of ointment, paint or lotion, but can in dilute solution be oral or as vaginal inserts (pessaries). The dye is also used to stain specimens for examination under a microscope. A non-proprietary antiseptic paint, used particularly to prepare skin for surgery, combines gentian violet with another dye, brilliant green.

▲ side-effects: rarely, there may be nausea and vomiting, with diarrhoea.

✚ warning: gentian violet is a dye: it stains clothes as well as skin.

Genticin (*Nicholas*) is a proprietary ANTIBIOTIC, available only on prescription, used to treat a number of serious gram-negative bacterial infections, but especially those of the urinary tract and of the skin. Produced in vials or ampoules for injection (in three strengths, the weakest under the name Genticin Paediatric), as a (water-miscible) cream or an (anhydrous greasy) ointment applied topically to treat skin infections, and as eye- or ear-drops, Genticin is a preparation of the aminoglycoside gentamicin.

▲/✚ side-effects/warning: *see* GENTAMICIN.

Genticin HC (*Nicholas*) is a proprietary compound ANTIBIOTIC, available only on prescription, used in the form of a cream and as an ointment to treat skin infections and to reduce the symptoms of allergic skin conditions. It is a preparation of the aminoglycoside ANTIBIOTIC gentamicin sulphate with the anti-inflammatory CORTICOSTEROID hydrocortisone acetate.

▲/✚ side-effects/warning: *see* GENTAMICIN.

Gentisone HC (*Nicholas*) is a proprietary compound ANTIBIOTIC, available only on prescription, used in the form of ear-drops to treat bacterial infections of the outer or middle ear. It is a preparation of the aminoglycoside gentamicin sulphate with the CORTICOSTEROID hydrocortisone acetate. Because of gentamicin's toxicity to the ear this preparation should not be used in cases where the ear drum is perforated.

▲/✚ side-effects/warning: *see* GENTAMICIN.

G

G

glutaraldehyde is a DISINFECTANT much like formaldehyde, but stronger and faster-acting. It is used mostly to sterilize medical and surgical equipment, but may alternatively be used therapeutically (in solution) to treat skin conditions such as warts (particularly verrucas on the soles of the feet) and to remove hard, dead skin.
➕ warning: effects of treatment are not always predictable. Skin treated may become sensitized.

Graneodin (*Squibb*) is a proprietary ANTIBIOTIC, available only on prescription, used to treat bacterial infections of the head and face, and particularly of the eye. Produced in the form of an ointment for topical application, Graneodin contains the aminoglycoside neomycin sulphate.
▲/➕ side-effects/warning: *see* NEOMYCIN.

Gregoderm (*Unigreg*) is a proprietary ANTIBIOTIC ANTIFUNGAL preparation, available only on prescription, used to treat inflammation of the skin in which infection is also present. Produced in the form of an ointment for topical application, Gregoderm is a compound of the aminoglycoside antibiotic neomycin sulphate and the antibiotic polymyxin B sulphate and the antifungal nystatin; together with the CORTICOSTEROID hydrocortisone.
▲/➕ side-effects/warning: *see* NEOMYCIN; NYSTATIN; POLYMYXIN B SULPHATE.

griseofulvin is a powerful ANTIFUNGAL drug that during treatment − which may be prolonged − is deposited selectively in the skin, hair and nails, and thus prevents further fungal invasion. It is most commonly used for large-scale infections, or to treat infections that prove intractable to other drugs, but can be used equally successfully on ringworm or localized tinea infections (such as athlete's foot). Administration is oral in the form of tablets or as a suspension.
▲ side-effects: there may be headache, with nausea and vomiting; some patients experience a sensitivity to light. Rarely, there may be a rash (which may be mild or serious).

G

✚ warning: griseofulvin should not be administered to
patients who suffer from liver failure or from
porphyria, or who are pregnant or taking oral
contraceptives. Avoid alcohol during the period of
treatment.
Related articles: FULCIN; GRISOVIN.

Grisovin (*Glaxo*) is a proprietary ANTIFUNGAL drug,
available only on prescription, used to treat infections of
the scalp, skin and nails. Produced in the form of tablets
(in two strengths), Grisovin is a preparation of the drug
griseofulvin. Treatment may be required to continue over
several weeks.
▲/✚ side-effects/warning: *see* GRISEOFULVIN.

Gynatren (*Cabot*) is a proprietary preparation of certain
bacilli that ordinarily reside in the alimentary tract and
vagina, consisting of a form of VACCINE used to treat
recurrent vaginal infections, particularly trichomaniasis.
Available only on prescription, it is produced in
ampoules for intramuscular injection, and administered
in 3 doses over four weeks.

Gyno-Daktarin (*Janssen*) is a series of proprietary
preparations of the ANTIFUNGAL drug miconazole nitrate,
used to treat yeast infections of the vagina or vulva (such
as thrush). All are available only on prescription. There
is an intravaginal cream (with its own applicator),
vaginal inserts (pessaries), coated tampons, an "ovule"
(which is a vaginal capsule, and marketed under the
name Gyno-Daktarin 1), and a Combipack combining the
cream and the pessaries.
▲/✚ side-effects/warning: *see* MICONAZOLE.

Gyno-Pevaryl (*Ortho-Cilag*) is a series of proprietary
preparations of the ANTIFUNGAL drug econazole nitrate,
used to treat yeast infections of the vagina or vulva (like
thrush). All are available only on prescription. There is a
cream for topical application to the anogenital area,
vaginal inserts (pessaries, in two formulations, one under

the name Gyno-Pevaryl 1), and a Combipack combining the cream and one or other formulation of the pessaries.

▲/✚ side-effects/warning: *see* ECONAZOLE NITRATE.

G

HBIG, or hepatitis B immunoglobulin, when injected or infused into the body, confers immediate immunity to the potentially dangerous effects of the disease caused by the hepatitis B virus. Prepared from the blood plasma of recent patients, it is used specifically to immunize personnel in medical laboratories and hospitals who may be infected, and to treat babies of mothers infected by the virus during pregnancy. In normal circumstances, however, immunization is with HEPATITIS B VACCINE.

H-B-Vax (*Merck, Sharp & Dohme*) is a proprietary form of HEPATITIS B VACCINE, available only on prescription, used on patients with a high risk of infection from the hepatitis B virus, mostly through contact with a carrier. Chemically, H-B-Vax consists of an inactivated hepatitis B virus surface antigen derived from the blood plasma of a human carrier and adsorbed on to alum in suspension. It is produced in vials for intramuscular injection; the usual regimen per patient is 3 doses, at intervals of one month and six months.

hepatitis B vaccine consists of an inactivated hepatitis B virus surface antigen derived from the blood plasma of a human carrier, or prepared biosynthetically, and adsorbed on to alum in suspension. It is used on patients with a high risk of infection from the hepatitis B virus mostly through contact with a carrier. Administration is by intramuscular injection in the arm or thigh; the usual regimen per patient is 3 doses, at intervals of one month and six months.

✚warning: vaccination does not guarantee the avoidance of infection: commonsense precautions against infection should still be observed in relation to known carriers.

Herpid (*WB Pharmaceuticals*) is a proprietary form of the ANTIVIRAL drug idoxuridine, prepared in a solution of dimethyl sulphoxide, used to treat skin infections by the viral organisms Herpes simplex (such as cold sores or genital sores) and Herpes zoster (shingles). Available only on prescription, Herpid is produced as a paint for topical application (with a brush).

✚ warning: see IDOXURIDINE.

Hewletts Antiseptic Cream (*Astra*) is a proprietary ANTISEPTIC cream for topical application on minor abrasions or burns. Available without prescription, it contains boric acid, hydrous wool fat and zinc oxide.

hexachlorophane is a powerful DISINFECTANT used on the skin, particularly of the face. In the form of a cream it is effective against scabies, and is a good substitute for soap in cases of acne or facial infection. It is also produced as a dusting-powder (which may help to prevent the onset of bedsores).

▲ side-effects: there are occasionally sensitivity reactions, and even more rarely an increased sensitivity to light.

✚ warning: hexachlorophane should not be used on areas of raw or abraded skin, and particularly not on raw areas of the skin of infants (in whom neural damage may occur). It is advisable to avoid using hexachlorophane routinely.
Related article: STER-ZAC.

hexamine is an ANTIBIOTIC that was formerly used to treat infections of the urinary tract. It is now generally considered to be too limited in its action − it limits only bacterial infection, requires the urine to be made to be acidic, and has many potentially unpleasant side-effects. Administration of its one proprietary form is oral, as tablets.

▲ side-effects: there may be bladder irritation, with frequent and painful urination, and possibly blood in the urine; there may also be gastrointestinal disturbances and rashes.

✚ warning: hexamine should not be administered to patients with impaired kidney or liver function, or who are dehydrated.
Related article: HIPREX.

Hibidil (*ICI*) is a proprietary non-prescription skin
DISINFECTANT used to treat wounds and burns, and to
provide asepsis during childbirth. Produced in the form
of a solution in sachets, for further dilution as required,
Hibidil is a preparation of chlorhexidine gluconate.
▲/✚ side-effects/warning: *see* CHLORHEXIDINE.

Hibiscrub (*ICI*) is a proprietary non-prescription
DISINFECTANT used instead of soap to wash skin and hands
before surgery. Produced in the form of a solution,
Hibiscrub is a preparation of chlorhexidine gluconate in
a surfactant liquid (a liquid with low surface tension,
like a detergent).
▲/✚ side-effects/warning: *see* CHLORHEXIDINE.

Hibisol (*ICI*) is a proprietary non-prescription
DISINFECTANT, used to treat minor wounds and burns on
the skin and hands. Produced in the form of a solution,
Hibisol is a preparation of chlorhexidine gluconate in
isopropyl alcohol solvent together with emollients.
▲/✚ side-effects/warning: *see* CHLORHEXIDINE.

Hibitane (*ICI*) is the name of a series or proprietary non-
prescription forms of DISINFECTANT, all based on solutions
of chlorhexidine gluconate or other chlorhexidine salts.
The standard form is that of a powder, used either to
prepare solutions of chlorhexidine or to create antiseptic
creams or powdered antiseptic compounds. There are two
solutions: Hibitane 5% Concentrate (for skin disinfection,
following further dilution in water or alcohol) and
Hibitane Gluconate 20% (for cavities and the bladder,
and to treat urethral infections). Hibitane Obstetric is a
water-miscible cream used to lubricate the vulva during
labour and childbirth. Another cream, Hibitane
Antiseptic, is used to treat minor wounds and burns by
topical application.
▲/✚ side-effects/warning: *see* CHLORHEXIDINE.

Hioxyl (*Quinoderm*) is a proprietary non-prescription
DISINFECTANT used to treat bedsores and leg ulcers, minor

wounds and burns. Produced in the form of a cream for topical application, Hioxyl is a preparation of the antiseptic HYDROGEN PEROXIDE.

Hiprex is a proprietary non-prescription ANTIBIOTIC used to treat infections of the urinary tract, and to prevent infection following urological surgery. Produced in the form of tablets, Hiprex is a compound of the now less commonly used drug hexamine together with hippuric acid (which renders the urine acidic enough for hexamine to be effective).

▲/✚ side-effects/warning: *see* HEXAMINE.

HNIG is an abbreviation for human normal immunoglobulin, an injection of which − incorporating antibodies in serum − confers immediate immunity to such diseases as infective hepatitis (hepatitis A virus), measles (rubeola), and to some degree at least rubella (German measles). Prepared from more than a thousand pooled donations of blood plasma, it is commonly given to patients at risk, such as infants who cannot tolerate vaccines which incorporate live (if attenuated) viruses. Administration is by intramuscular injection or occasionally by intravenous infusion.

✚ warning: HNIG should not be administered within 2 weeks following vaccination with live viruses, or within 3 months before vaccination with live viruses is to be given (except in specific circumstances relating to the likelihood of convulsions in patients known to be at risk from them).

HTIG is an abbreviation for human tetanus immunoglobulin, a specific form of immunoglobulin (antibodies in serum), used mostly as an added precaution to treat patients with contaminated wounds. (It is generally only a precautionary measure because almost everybody today has established immunity through vaccination from an early age, and vaccination is in any case readily available for those at risk.) Administration is by intramuscular injection. It is available only on prescription.

Humotet (*Wellcome*) is a proprietary preparation of anti-tetanus immunoglobulin (HTIG), available only on prescription, used mostly as an added precaution to treat patients with contaminated wounds. (It is generally only a precautionary measure because almost everybody today has established immunity through vaccination from an early age, and vaccination is in any case readily available for those at risk.) It is produced in vials for intramuscular injection.

hydrogen peroxide is a general DISINFECTANT used in solution and as a cream to cleanse and deodorize wounds and ulcers, to clean ears in the form of ear-drops, and as a mouth wash and gargle for oral hygiene. Some preparations available require further dilution: a 6% solution is the maximum concentration recommended for use on the skin. Stronger solutions will bleach fabric. *Related article:* HIOXYL.

Idoxene (*Spodefell*) is a proprietary ANTIVIRAL eye ointment, available only on prescription, used to treat local viral infections, particularly of herpes simplex. It is a preparation of idoxuridine.

▲/✚ side-effects/warning: *see* IDOXURIDINE.

idoxuridine is an ANTIVIRAL drug used primarily in very mild solution to treat infections caused by herpes viruses in and around the mouth or eye. In a solution of dimethyl sulphoxide, however, it is alternatively used to treat herpes zoster skin infections. It inhibits the multiplication of the virus by interfering with viral DNA synthesis. Administration is as a paint for topical application, as eye-drops or as eye ointment.

✚ warning: because idoxuridine contains iodine, treatment may cause initial irritation and/or stinging. *Related articles:* HERPID; IDOXENE; IDURIDIN; KERECID; OPHTHALMADINE.

Iduridin (*Ferring*) is a proprietary ANTIVIRAL drug, available only on prescription, used to treat infections of the skin by herpes simplex (cold sores, fever sores) or by herpes zoster (shingles). Produced in the form of a lotion or paint, for topical application either with a dropper or its own applicator, Iduridin is a solution of idoxuridine in the organic solvent dimethyl sulphoxide (DMSO).

✚ warning: see IDOXURIDINE.

Ilosone (*Dista*) is a proprietary macrolide ANTIBIOTIC, available only on prescription, used to treat many serious infections (such as legionnaires' disease and inflammation of the prostate gland) and to prevent others (such as diphtheria or whooping cough), but more commonly in the treatment of infections of the upper respiratory tract or of infected wounds, especially in patients who are allergic to penicillin-type antibiotics. Produced in the form of capsules, tablets, and as a suspension (in two strengths, the stronger under the name Ilosone Suspension Forte) for dilution (the potency of the suspension once diluted is retained for 14 days),

Ilosone in every form is a preparation of erythromycin estolate.

▲/✚ side-effects/warning: *see* ERYTHROMYCIN.

*imidazoles are a group of broad-spectrum ANTIFUNGAL drugs active against most fungi and yeasts. The most common conditions that they are used to treat are vaginal infections (such as candidiasis, or thrush) and infections of the skin surface and mucous membranes, the hair and the nails. Best known and most used imidazoles include clotrimazole, miconazole, ketoconazole and econazole. Miconazole and ketoconazole may be used systemically, although the latter can cause serious toxicity to the liver (hepatoxicity) and systemic use should be reserved for serious infections.

see CLOTRIMAZOLE; ECONAZOLE; KETOCONAZOLE; MICONAZOLE.

*immunization against specific diseases is effected by either of two means. Active immunity is conferred by vaccination, in which live antigens that have been rendered harmless (attenuated), or dead ones (inactivated), are injected into the bloodstream so that the body's own defence mechanisms are required to deal with them (by manufacturing antibodies) and with anything like them that they encounter again. This method gives long-lasting but impermanent protection (and there is a slight risk of allergic reaction or toxic effect). Passive immunity is conferred by the injection of a quantity of blood serum already containing antibodies (immunoglobulins), or of the purified, specific immunoglobulins themselves; this method gives immediate but short-lived protection, and carries the risk of sensitizing the individual to future exposure to similar injections.

see IMMUNOGLOBULINS; VACCINES.

*immunocompromised is a term that refers to a host whose immune defences are very much lower than normal due to either a congenital or acquired condition. The commonest deficiencies are: of the white cells, neutrophils, which are the first line of defence in acute infections; of the white cells, macrophages, and T lymphocytes, which are involved in cell-mediated killing of foreign or "parasitized" host cells; and of the antibodies, which neutralize and bind to foreign antigens. Examples of immunocompromised hosts are patients receiving immunosuppressant drugs to prevent rejection of transplanted organs. Individuals suffering from leukaemia, or being treated with high doses of cytotoxic drugs to treat cancer, will also be immunocompromised, as will individuals with AIDS. In any of these circumstances "opportunistic" infections are apt to occur where microbes which normally pose little threat to the healthy become highly invasive and pose a serious threat. Prophylaxis with antibiotics may be required, and once infections are established they are much more difficult to eradicate even with vigorous antibiotic treatment.

*immunoglobulins are proteins of a specific structure, which act as antibodies in the bloodstream. Created in response to the presence of a specific antigen, immunoglobulins circulate with the blood to give systemic defence and protection as part of the immune system. Immunoglobulin deficiences are often associated with increased risk of infection. Classified according to a differentiation of class and function, immunoglobulins may be administered therapeutically by injection or infusion to confer immediate (passive) immunity.
see IMMUNIZATION.
Related article: HNIG.

Imperacin (*ICI*) is a proprietary broad-spectrum ANTIBIOTIC, available only on prescription, used to treat serious infections by bacteria and other micro-organisms (such as chlamydia and rickettsia), and to relieve severe acne. Produced in the form of tablets, Imperacin is a preparation of the TETRACYCLINE oxytetracycline dihydrate. It is not recommended for children.
▲/✚ side-effects/warning: *see* OXYTETRACYCLINE.

Imunovir (*Burgess*) is a proprietary preparation of the

ANTIVIRAL drug inosine pranobex, available only on prescription, used to treat herpes simplex infections and warts in mucous membranes and adjacent skin, particularly in or on the genitalia. It is produced in the form of tablets.

▲/✚ side-effects/warning: *see* INOSINE PRANOBEX.

*influenza vaccines are recommended only for persons at high risk of catching known strains of influenza. This is because the influenza viruses A and B are constantly changing in physical form, and antibodies manufactured in the body to deal with one strain at one time will have no effect at all on the same strain at another time. Consequently, it is only possible to provide vaccine for any single strain once it has already shown itself to be endemic. Moreover, during times when no influenza strain is endemic, vaccination against influenza is positively discouraged. The World Health Organisation makes an annual recommendation on the strains of virus for which stocks of vaccine should be prepared. Administration is by injection of surface-antigen vaccine: a single dose for adults (unless the specific strain is in the process of changing again and two slightly different doses are required), two doses over 5 weeks or so for children. As the vaccines are prepared from virus strains grown in chicken embryos, the vaccines should not be given to individuals known to be sensitive to eggs. *Related articles:* FLUVIRIN; INFLUVAC SUB-UNIT; MFV-JECT.

Influvac Sub-unit (*Duphar*) is the name of a series of proprietary flu vaccines consisting of inactivated surface antigens of the influenza virus. None is recommended for children aged under 4 years.

▲ side-effects: rarely, there is local reaction together with headache and high temperature.

✚ warning: like any flu vaccine, Influvac Sub-unit cannot control epidemics and should be used only — in what seems to be the appropriate strain — to treat people who are at high risk: the elderly, patients with cardiovascular problems, and medical staff. Influvac

Sub-unit should not be administered to patients who are allergic to egg or chicken protein (in which vaccine viruses are cultured), or who are pregnant.

inosine pranobex is an ANTIVIRAL drug introduced recently, used primarily to treat herpes simplex infections in mucous membranes and adjacent skin, particularly in or on the genitalia; it is also effective in removing warts in similar areas. Administered in the form of tablets, it works partly by increasing the local activity of the body's own immune system.

▲ side-effects: uric acid levels rise in the blood and in the urine.

✚ warning: inosine pranobex should not be administered to patients with impaired kidney function or high blood levels of uric acid (as with gout).

Related article: IMUNOVIR.

Instillagel (*Rimmer*) is a proprietary compound preparation, available only on prescription, in the form of a water-miscible gel produced in disposable syringes that combines a local anaesthetic with a powerful disinfectant. It is used primarily to treat painful inflammations of the urethra: the compound is instilled into the urethra after external cleansing. But it may also be used to disinfect and lubricate medical equipment following such procedures as catheterization and cystoscopy. The anaesthetic constituent is lignocaine hydrochloride; the major antiseptic constituent is chlorhexidine gluconate.

▲/✚ side-effects/warning: *see* CHLORHEXIDINE.

*interferons are proteins produced in tiny quantities by cells infected by a virus; they have the ability to inhibit further growth by the virus. Genetic engineering, including the use of bacteria as host cells, has enabled interferons to be mass-produced − but they have not turned out to be the ultimate weapon against viruses that it was thought they would be. But because they have specific and complex effects on cells, cell function and immunity, interferons are now undergoing trials in the treatment of cancers (particularly lymphomas and certain solid tumours).

▲ side-effects: symptoms of severe fever are common; there may also be lethargy and/or depression. The blood-producing capacity of the bone marrow may be reduced. Some patients experience high or low blood pressure, and heartbeat irregularities.

✚ warning: regular blood counts are essential during treatment, particularly to check on levels of white blood cells that contribute to the immune system.

Intraglobin (*Biotest Folex*) is a proprietary preparation of human normal IMMUNOGLOBULIN (HNIG) as a powder for reconstitution in solvent, used in infusion to confer immediate immunity to diseases such as hepatitis A virus, measles (rubeola) and at least to some degree rubella (German measles), particularly in patients who for one reason or another cannot tolerate the administration of live (though attenuated) viruses in vaccination therapies. Intraglobin is also used to provide some form of immunity in patients born with immunodeficient conditions. It is available only on prescription.

✚ warning: see HNIG.

iodine is an element required in small quantities in the diet for healthy growth and development. More mundanely, iodine is still commonly used as an ANTISEPTIC (either as aqueous iodine solution or as POVIDINE-IODINE).

▲ side-effects: there may be sensitivity reactions.

Iodosorb (*Stuart*) is a proprietary ANTISEPTIC powder, available only on prescription, and is an absorbent material that cleans, dries and removes dead skin from leg ulcers and open bedsores. Applied to the site, the powder should be covered with a sterile dressing changed daily. Iodosorb powder is based on a form of iodine, and is produced in sachets.

Ipral (*Squibb*) is a proprietary ANTIBIOTIC, available only on prescription, used to treat infections of the upper respiratory tract (particularly bronchitis and bronchial pneumonia) and of the urinary tract. Produced in the form of tablets (in two strengths) and as a sugar-free suspension for children (under the trade name Ipral Paediatric) for dilution (the potency of the suspension once diluted is retained for 14 days), Ipral is a preparation of the antibacterial drug trimethoprim.

▲/✚ side-effects/warning: *see* TRIMETHOPRIM.

isoconazole is an ANTIFUNGAL drug, one of the IMIDAZOLES, used particularly to treat fungal infections of the vagina and anogenital area. Administration is in the form of a cream or as vaginal tablets (pessaries), usually as a single-dose treatment. It is not recommended for children.

▲ side-effects: there may be local irritation, and even a temporary burning sensation.

Related article: TRAVOGYN.

isoniazid is an ANTITUBERCULAR drug used, as is normal in the treatment of tuberculosis, in combination with other antibacterial drugs to defeat bacterial resistance. It is also administered to prevent the contraction of tuberculosis by close associates of an infected patient. Administration is oral in the form of tablets or as a non-proprietary elixir, or by injection.

▲ side-effects: there may be nausea with vomiting. High dosage may lead to sensitivity reactions, including a rash, and in susceptible patients to a peripheral neuritis leading to loss of sensation in the hands and feet, convulsions and/or psychotic episodes.

✚ warning: isoniazid should not be administered to patients with liver disease induced by drug treatment; it should be administered with caution to those with impaired kidney or liver function, epilepsy or alcoholism, or who are lactating.

Related article: RIMIFON.

Isopto (*Alcon*) is a series of proprietary preparations of various drugs, all available only on prescription. Each preparation of Isopto is used in the form of eye-drops used variously to treat infections of the eye such as conjunctivitis and blepharitis, to treat glaucoma, and to facilitate inspection of the eye. The range includes the preparation Isopto Cetamide (comprising the sulphonamide sulphacetamide sodium and the synthetic tear medium hypromellose).

▲/✚ side-effects/warning: *see* PRIMARY CONSTITUENTS LISTED ABOVE.

itraconazole is a broad-spectrum ANTIFUNGAL drug of the triazole family. Orally absorbed, it is used to treat resistant forms of candidiasis (thrush, or moniliasis) of the vagina or vulva and for dermatophyte infections of the skin, or finger-nails by tinea organisms, including ringworm and athlete's foot. Itraconazole is broken down in the liver and should therefore not be given to individuals with impaired liver function.

▲ side-effects: nausea and gastrointestinal disturbance causing abdominal pains and dyspepsia may occur; there may also be headaches.

✚ warning: itraconazole should not be used with a patient with impaired liver function, in pregnancy or when lactating.

ivermectin is an ANTIFUNGAL drug that is not available in the United Kingdom. Ivermectin is used to treat the tropical disease onchocerciasis − infestation by the filarial worm-parasite *Onchocerca volvulus*. The destruction of the worms, however, releases antigens into the bloodstream and causes an allergic response, generally requiring the simultaneous administration of antihistamines or CORTICOSTEROIDS to control it. More than one course of treatment with ivermectin may be necessary to deal with the infestation.

▲ side-effects: headache, with nausea and vomiting, is not uncommon; the dermatitis associated with onchocerciasis may temporarily be aggravated, as may any associated conjunctivitis or other eye inflammation.

➕ warning: close medical supervision is essential during treatment.

Kabiglobulin (*KabiVitrum*) is a proprietary preparation of human normal immunoglobulin (HNIG), part of the plasma of the blood that is directly concerned with immunity. Administered by intramuscular injection, Kabiglobulin is used to protect patients at risk from contact with hepatitis A virus, measles (rubeola) or at least to some degree rubella (German measles), or to replace some measure of immunity in patients who have suffered serious shock (as for example with large-scale burns).

✚warning: *see* HNIG.

kanamycin is a broad-spectrum ANTIBIOTIC of the aminoglycoside family, with activity against gram-positive bacteria but used primarily against serious infections caused by gram-negative bacteria. It is not orally absorbed and is therefore given by injection or infusion for the treatment of, for example, septicaemia, meningitis and infections of the heart (usually in conjunction with penicillin), the kidney and the prostate gland. Because of its toxicity to the ear (ototoxicity) potentially resulting in deafness, and its toxicity to the kidney (nephrotoxicity), treatment should be limited in duration. Because of the relatively frequent occurrence of bacterial resistance in some coliform bacteria, kanamycin has largely been replaced by gentamicin.

▲side-effects: prolonged or high dosage may be damaging to the ear, causing deafness and balance disorders; treatment must be discontinued if this occurs; there may also be reversible kidney damage.

✚warning: kanamycin should not be administered to patients who are pregnant or who suffer from myasthenia gravis. It should be administered with caution to those with Parkinsonism. As the drug is excreted by the kidney, great care must be taken in patients with impaired kidney function. In such cases, and/or where dosage is high or prolonged, regular checks on kanamycin concentrations in the blood must be carried out.

Related article: KANNASYN.

Kannasyn (*Winthrop*) is a proprietary form of the aminoglycoside ANTIBIOTIC kanamycin sulphate, available only on prescription, used to treat serious bacterial infections. It is produced in the form of solution and as powder for reconstitution, in both cases for injection.
▲/✚ side-effects/warning: *see* KANAMYCIN.

K

Kefadol (*Dista*) is a proprietary ANTIBIOTIC, available only on prescription, used to treat both gram-positive and gram-negative bacterial infections. It may be used to prevent infections following abdominal surgery. Produced in the form of a powder for reconstitution as injections, Kefadol is a compound of the CEPHALOSPORIN cephamandole with sodium carbonate.
▲/✚ side-effects/warning: *see* CEPHAMANDOLE.

Keflex (*Lilly*) is a proprietary ANTIBIOTIC, available only on prescription, used to treat sensitive bacterial infections. Produced in the form of capsules (in two strengths), tablets (in two strengths) and a suspension (for dilution, in two strengths), Keflex is a preparation of the orally active CEPHALOSPORIN cephalexin.
▲/✚ side-effects/warning: *see* CEPHALEXIN.

Keflin (*Lilly*) is a proprietary ANTIBIOTIC, available only on prescription, used to treat sensitive bacterial infections, but also to prevent infection following surgery. Produced in the form of powder for reconstitution as injections, Keflin is a preparation of the CEPHALOSPORIN cephalothin.
▲/✚ side-effects/warning: *see* CEPHALOTHIN.

Kefzol (*Lilly*) is a proprietary ANTIBIOTIC, available only on prescription, used to treat bacterial infections, but also to provide freedom from infection during surgery. Produced in the form of powder for reconstitution as injections, Kefzol is a preparation of the CEPHALOSPORIN CEPHAZOLIN.
▲/✚ side-effects/warning: *see* CEPHAZOLIN.

Kelfizine W (*Farmitalia Carlo Erba*) is a proprietary ANTIBIOTIC, available only on prescription, used primarily

to treat chronic bronchitis and infections of the urinary tract. Produced in the form of tablets, Kelfizine W is a preparation of the SULPHONAMIDE sulfametopyrazine.
▲/✚ side-effects/warning: *see* SULFAMETOPYRAZINE.

Kemicetine (*Farmitalia Carlo Erba*) is a proprietary broad-spectrum ANTIBIOTIC, available only on prescription. Produced in the form of powder for reconstitution as injections, Kemicetine is a preparation of the powerful drug chloramphenicol which, because of its potential toxicity, is generally used systemically only to treat life-threatening infections.
▲/✚ side-effects/warning: *see* CHLORAMPHENICOL.

Kerecid (*Smith, Kline & French*) is a proprietary preparation, available only on prescription, used to treat herpes simplex infections of the eye. Containing a mild solution of the antiviral agent idoxuridine, it is produced in the form of eye-drops (with polyvinyl alcohol) for use during the day, and eye ointment for use overnight.
✚ warning: *see* IDOXURIDINE.

ketoconazole is a broad-spectrum ANTIFUNGAL agent, an imidazole that is effective when taken orally, used to treat deep-seated fungal infections (mycoses) or superficial ones that have not responded to other treatment. In particular, ketoconazole is used to treat resistant candidiasis (thrush, or moniliasis) and serious dermatophytic infections of the skin or fingernails.
▲ side-effects: liver damage may occur − and to a serious extent; rarely there may be an itching skin rash, or nausea.
✚ warning: ketoconazole should not be administered to patients who have impaired liver function, or who are pregnant. Because it may cause serious liver toxicity it should not be used for minor fungal infections.
Related article: NIZORAL.

Ladropen (*Berk*) is a proprietary ANTIBIOTIC, available only on prescription, used to treat gram-positive bacterial infections of the skin and of the ear, nose and throat, and especially staphylococcal infections that prove to be resistant to penicillin. Produced in the form of capsules (in two strengths), Ladropen is a preparation of flucloxacillin. It is not suitable for children.

▲/✚ side-effects/warning: *see* FLUCLOXACILLIN.

Laratrim (*Lagap*) is a proprietary broad-spectrum ANTIBIOTIC, available only on prescription, used to treat infections of the urinary tract, the sinuses or the middle ear, an inflamed prostate gland, or exacerbated chronic bronchitis. Produced in the form of tablets (in two strengths, the stronger under the name Laratrim Forte) and as a suspension (in two strengths, Laratrim Paediatric Suspension and Laratrim Adult Suspension), Laratrim is a compound combination of the drug trimethoprim and the SULPHONAMIDE sulphamethoxazole.

▲/✚ side-effects/warning: *see* CO-TRIMOXAZOLE.

latamoxef disodium is a third-generation CEPHALOSPORIN ANTIBIOTIC used to treat many bacterial infections. Unlike early cephalosporins it has effective activity against many gram-negative bacteria. Administration is by injection.

✚ warning: latamoxef should be used with caution in patients taking anticoagulants and with bleeding tendencies; it should be administered with caution to those known to have penicillin sensitivity, and not at all to those with known sensitivity to cephalosporins. Dosage should be reduced in patients with impaired liver function.

▲ side-effects: there may be hypersensitivity reactions, effects on the white cells of the blood (on which it may have an anticoagulating influence). Rarely there is diarrhoea.

Related article: MOXALACTAM.

Ledermycin (*Lederle*) is a proprietary ANTIBIOTIC, available only on prescription, used to treat infections of soft tissues, particularly of the upper respiratory tract. Produced in the form of tablets (in two strengths, the stronger under the name Ledermycin Tablets), Ledermycin is a preparation of the TETRACYCLINE DEMECLOCYCLINE HYDROCHLORIDE.

▲/✚ side-effects/warning: *see* DEMECLOCYCLINE HYDROCHLORIDE.

levamisole is an ANTHELMINTIC drug used specifically to treat infestation by roundworms. Effective, it is also well tolerated and side-effects are rare. Occasionally there may be mild nausea.

Lincocin (*Upjohn*) is a proprietary ANTIBIOTIC, available only on prescription, used to treat serious infections of the tissues and bones (particularly infections that prove to be resistant to penicillin). Produced in the form of capsules, as a syrup for dilution (the potency of the syrup once diluted is retained for 14 days) and in ampoules for injection, Lincocin is a preparation of lincomycin.

▲/✚ side-effects/warning: *see* LINCOMYCIN.

lincomycin is an ANTIBIOTIC that is now used less commonly than it once was (because of side-effects) to treat infections of bones and joints, and peritonitis (inflammation of the peritoneal lining of the abdominal cavity due to gram-positive cocci or anaerobic bacteria). Administration is oral in the form of capsules and as a dilute syrup, or by injection or infusion.

▲ side-effects: if diarrhoea or other symptoms of colitis appear during treatment, administration must be halted at once (*see below*). There may be nausea and vomiting.

✚ warning: lincomycin should not be administered to patients suffering from diarrhoea; if diarrhoea or other symptoms of colitis appear during treatment, administration must be halted at once. This is because lincomycin's disturbance of the balance of intestinal micro-organisms disposes towards a superinfection with the anaerobic bacterium *Clostridium difficile*, which causes a severe pseudomembranous colitis

(particularly in adult/elderly females). It should be administered with caution to patients with impaired liver or kidney function.
Related article: LINCOCIN.

lindane, or gamma benzene hexachloride, is a drug used to treat parasitic infestation by lice (pediculosis) or by itch-mites (scabies) on the skin surface, particularly under the hair. However, strains of head-lice resistant to lindane have recently emerged, and the drug is now not recommended for use on the scalp. Administration is topical in the form of a lotion or a shampoo, to be left wet as long as possible.
▲ side-effects: side-effects are rare, but a few patients suffer minor skin irritation.
✚ warning: keep lindane away from the eyes.
Related articles: ESODERM; LOREXANE; QUELLADA.

Locabiotal (*Servier*) is a proprietary ANTIBIOTIC, available only on prescription, used to treat infection and inflammation in the nose and throat. Produced in an aerosol with a nose and mouth adaptor, Locabiotal is a preparation of fusafungine. It is not recommended for children aged under 3 years.

Locorten-Vioform (*Ciba*) is a proprietary ANTIBACTERIAL and ANTIFUNGAL, available only on prescription, used to treat mild infections of the outer ear. Produced in the form of ear-drops, Locorten-Vioform is a compound of clioquinol and the minor CORTICOSTEROID flumethasone pivalate.
▲/✚ side-effects/warning: *see* CLIOQUINOL.

Lorexane (*Care*) is a proprietary non-prescription preparation of the parasiticidal drug lindane, used to treat infestation of the skin of the trunk and limbs by itch-mites (scabies) or by lice (pediculosis). It is produced in the form of a water-miscible cream and (under the name Lorexane No. 3) as a shampoo.
▲/✚ side-effects/warning: *see* LINDANE.

Lugacin (*Lagap*) is a proprietary ANTIBIOTIC, available only on prescription, used to treat serious gram-negative infections in specific organs, such as meningitis. Produced in ampoules for injection, Lugacin is a preparation of the aminoglycoside gentamicin.
✚warning: *see* GENTAMICIN.

lymecycline is a broad-spectrum ANTIBIOTIC, one of the TETRACYCLINES, used to treat infections of many kinds. Administration is oral in the form of capsules.
▲ side-effects: there may be nausea and vomiting, with diarrhoea. Some patients experience a sensitivity to light. Rarely, there are allergic reactions.
✚warning: lymecycline should not be administered to patients with kidney failure, who are pregnant, or who are aged under 12 years. It should be administered with caution to those who are lactating, or who have impaired liver function.
Related article: TETRALYSAL.

Macrodantin (*Norwich Eaton*) is a proprietary ANTIBIOTIC, available only on prescription, used to treat infections of the urinary tract. It works by interfering with the DNA of specific bacteria. Produced in the form of capsules (in two strengths), Macrodantin is a preparation of the antibacterial nitrofurantoin. It is not recommended for children aged under 30 months.

▲/➕ side-effects/warning: *see* NITROFURANTOIN.

Madribon (*Roche*) is a proprietary ANTIBACTERIAL, available only on prescription, used to treat a number of bacterial infections — of the upper respiratory tract, of the ear, nose or throat, the skin, but particularly of the urinary tract. Produced in the form of tablets, Madribon is a preparation of the sulphonamide sulphadimethoxine. It is not recommended for children aged under 2 years.

▲/➕ side-effects/warning: *see* SULPHADIMETHOXINE.

mafenide is an ANTIBIOTIC, a SULPHONAMIDE used (as mafenide propionate) to treat infections in and around the eye, and (as mafenide acetate) to treat infectious burns. Administration is thus both in solution as eye-drops, and as a cream.

▲ side-effects: acid levels in the body may become high.
➕ warning: mafenide acetate should be administered with caution to patients with respiratory problems.

Magnapen (*Beecham*) is a proprietary compound ANTIBIOTIC, available only on prescription, used to treat severe infection where the causative organism has not been identified, but gram-positive staphylococcal infection is suspected, or where penicillin-resistant bacterial infection is probable. Produced in the form of capsules, as a syrup (under the name Magnapen Syrup), as a powder for reconstitution as a syrup, and in vials for injections (under the name Magnapen Injection), Magnapen is a preparation of the broad-spectrum penicillin-like antibiotic ampicillin together with the anti-staphylococcal antibiotic flucloxacillin.

▲/➕ side-effects/warning: *see* AMPICILLIN; FLUCLOXACILLIN.

Malarivon (*Wallace*) is a proprietary ANTIMALARIAL drug, available only on prescription, used both to prevent and to treat malaria. Produced in the form of an elixir, Malarivon is a preparation of the powerful drug chloroquine.

▲/✚ side-effects/warning: *see* CHLOROQUINE.

malathion is an insecticidal drug used to treat infestations by lice (pediculosis) or by itch-mites (scabies). Administration is topical in the form of a lotion or a shampoo, but treatment should not take place more than once a week for more than three weeks in succession. Some of the proprietary forms are highly inflammable.
✚ warning: avoid contact with the eyes.

   Related articles: DERBAC-M; PRIODERM; SULEO-M.

Maloprim (*Wellcome*) is a proprietary ANTIMALARIAL drug, available only on prescription, used to prevent travellers to tropical areas from contracting the disease. Produced in the form of tablets, Maloprim is a compound of the sulphone dapsone together with the catalytic enzyme-inhibitor pyrimethamine (which is particularly useful in relation to malarial strains resistant to chloroquine). It is commonly used in conjunction with chloroquine. Treatment is weekly, not daily, but must be continued for at least 4 weeks after the patient leaves the tropical area.

▲/✚ side-effects/warning: *see* DAPSONE; PYRIMETHAMINE.

Mansil is a proprietary form of the ANTHELMINTIC drug oxaminiquine, used to treat schistosomiasis (bilharziasis).
see OXAMINIQUINE.

Manusept (*Hough/Hoseason*) is a proprietary non-prescription ANTISEPTIC, used particularly as a hand cleanser prior to surgery, but also to moisturize dry skin. It consists of a preparation of the alcohol-based disinfectant triclosan in very mild solution.

mebendazole is an ANTHELMINTIC drug used in the treatment of infections by roundworm, threadworm, whipworm and hookworm. A powerful drug generally well tolerated, it is the treatment of choice for patients of all ages over 2 years.

▲ side-effects: side-effects are uncommon, but there may be diarrhoea and abdominal pain.

✚ warning: mebendazole should not be administered to patients who are aged under 2 years; it should be administered with caution to those who are pregnant. *Related article:* VERMOX.

mecillinam is a penicillin-type ANTIBIOTIC but with a different mechanism of action to most of the penicillins. Unlike the classic penicillins it has little activity against gram-positive bacteria but is active against some gram-negative bacteria. It is used primarily to treat sensitive urinary tract infections and systemic salmonella infections. Administration is in the form of injection.

▲ side-effects: there may be sensitivity reactions ranging from a minor rash to urticaria and joint pains, and (occasionally) to high temperature or anaphylactic shock.

✚ warning: mecillinam should not be administered to patients known to be allergic to penicillins; it should be administered with caution to those with impaired kidney function. Prolonged treatment requires regular checks on liver and kidney function. *Related article:* SELEXIDIN.

Mefoxin (*Merck, Sharp & Dohme*) is a proprietary broad-spectrum ANTIBIOTIC, available only on prescription, used to treat bacterial infections and to ensure asepsis during surgery. Produced in the form of a powder for reconstitution as a medium for injection, Mefoxin is a preparation of the CEPHALOSPORIN cefoxitin.

▲/✚ side-effects/warning: *see* CEFOXITIN.

Megaclor (*Pharmax*) is a proprietary ANTIBIOTIC, available only on prescription, used to treat infections of soft tissues, particularly of the upper respiratory tract, and to relieve the symptoms of acne. Produced in the form of

capsules, Megaclor is a preparation of the TETRACYCLINE clomocycline sodium. It is not recommended for children.
▲/✚ side-effects/warning: *see* CLOMOCYCLINE SODIUM.

Mengivax (A&C) (*Merieux*) is a VACCINE designed to give protection against the organism meningococcus, which can cause serious infection including meningitis. It may be indicated for travellers intending to go to parts of the world where the risk of meningococcal infection is much higher than in the United Kingdom, e.g. parts of Africa. It may be given to adults and children aged over 18 months.

mepacrine hydrochloride is a drug with ANTIPROTOZOAL properties used primarily to treat infection by the intestinal protozoon *Giardia lamblia*; giardiasis occurs throughout the world, particularly in children, and is contracted by eating contaminated food. It has largely been superseded by METRONIDAZOLE. Mepacrine can also be used to assist in the treatment of most forms of malaria.

Merieux Inactivated Rabies Vaccine is a proprietary preparation of rabies VACCINE with two uses. Firstly, it may be used prophylactically to prevent individuals who might be at risk from contracting rabies should they be bitten by a rabid animal. Secondly, it may be used after an unvaccinated individual has been bitten by a suspected rabid animal to prevent growth of the virus. It is the only vaccine which can be used in this way, post exposure. The success of such treatment is related to how soon after the bite the injections of the vaccine are given. Ideally they should be on days 0, 3, 7, 14, 30 and 100. Available only on prescription, the vaccine is of a type known as human diploid cell vaccine and has no known contra-indications. It is freeze-dried and produced in vials with a diluent for injection.
see RABIES VACCINE.

Merieux Tetavax (*Merieux*) is a proprietary preparation of tetanus VACCINE, formed of tetanus toxin (i.e. a toxoid vaccine) adsorbed on to a mineral carrier (in the form of aluminium hydroxide) and produced in syringes and in vials for injection.

see TETANUS VACCINE.

Meruvax II (*Morson*) is a proprietary VACCINE against German measles (rubella) in the form of a solution containing live but attenuated viruses of the Wistar RA27/3 strain. Available only on prescription, it is administered in the form of an injection.

see RUBELLA VACCINE.

methicillin is an ANTIBIOTIC of the penicillin family which was the first of the type to be resistant to the penicillinase enzyme secreted by penicillin-resistant strains of *Staphylococcus aureus*. It has been largely superseded by orally-active penicillinase-resistant penicillins, e.g. flucloxacillin. Methicillin has to be given by injection or infusion. In recent years the occurrence of methicillin-resistant strains of Staphylococcus has created major problems in hospitals throughout the world.

▲ side-effects: there may be sensitivity reactions ranging from a minor rash to urticaria and joint pains, and (occasionally) to fever or anaphylactic shock.

✚ warning: methicillin should not be administered to patients known to the allergic to penicillins; it should be administered with caution to those with impaired kidney function.

Related article: CELBENIN.

metriphonate is an organo-phosphorus compound that destroys the blood fluke *Schistosoma haematobium*, which causes a form of bilharzia that is common in North Africa and the Middle East. The disease is contracted by bathing in water contaminated by the larvae of the flukes; adult flukes of this species infest the veins of the bladder, ureter and other pelvic organs, causing severe inflammation. Administration is oral in three doses over four weeks. The drug has largely been superseded by PRAZIQUANTEL.

Metrolyl (*Lagap*) is a proprietary drug with ANTIBIOTIC and ANTIPROTOZOAL properties. Available only on prescription it is used to treat many forms of infection including those caused by bacteria (such as non-specific vaginitis), and by protozoa. Produced in the form of tablets (in two strengths), as anal suppositories (in two strengths), and in solution for intravenous infusion, Metrolyl is a preparation of metronidazole.

▲/✚ side-effects/warning: *see* METRONIDAZOLE.

metronidazole is an ANTIMICROBIAL with ANTIBIOTIC and ANTIPROTOZOAL properties. Its antibiotic spectrum is narrow, being limited to activity against strictly anaerobic bacteria. It acts by interfering with DNA replication. The other group of microbes it is active against are the protozoa, specifically *Entamoeba histolytica* (causes amoebic dysentery), *Giardia lamblia* (causes giardiasis, an infection of the small intestine) and *Trichomonas vaginalis* (causes vaginitis). Resistance is rare and this drug has radically improved the success of treating anaerobic infections such as may be found in peritonitis, pelvic abscess, brain abscess and wound infections. One reason for its activity in such situations is its ability to penetrate and remain effective in the presence of pus. Administration is oral in the form of tablets or a suspension, topical in the form of anal suppositories, or by injection or infusion.

▲ side-effects: these are uncommon — but there may be nausea and vomiting, with drowsiness, headache and gastrointestinal disturbances; gastrointestinal effects may be reduced by taking the drug during or after food. Some patients experience a discoloration of the urine. Prolonged treatment may eventually give rise to neuromuscular disorders or even seizures reminiscent of epilepsy with high doses.

✚ warning: metronidazole should not be taken regularly on a high-dosage basis. It should be administered with caution to patients with impaired liver function, or who are pregnant or lactating. During treatment patients must avoid alcohol consumption (the presence

of alcohol in the body during treatment gives rise to most unpleasant side-effects).
Related articles: FLAGYL; FLAGYL COMPAK; FLAGYL S; METROLYL; NIDAZOL; ZADSTAT.

metronidazole benzoate is the form in which the ANTIBIOTIC metronidazole is administered in a suspension. *see* METRONIDAZOLE.

Mevillin-L (*Evans*) is a proprietary VACCINE against measles (rubeola), available only on prescription. It is a powdered preparation of live but attenuated measles viruses for administration within a diluent by injection.
▲ side-effects: there may be inflammation at the site of injection. Rarely, there may be high temperature, cough and sore throat, a rash, swelling of the lymph glands and/or pain in the joints.
✚ warning: mevillin-L should not be administered to patients with any infection, particularly tuberculosis; who are allergic to eggs (the viruses are cultured in chick embryo tissue); who have known immune-system abnormalities; who are pregnant; who are hypersensitive to neomycin or polymyxin; or who are already taking corticosteroid drugs, cytotoxic drugs or are undergoing radiating treatment. It should be administered with caution to those with epilepsy or any other condition potentially involving convulsive fits.

mezlocillin is a derivative of the broad-spectrum penicillin-type ANTIBIOTIC ampicillin that has increased activity against some important gram-negative bacteria such as *Klessiella* and *Pseudomonas*. Administration is by injection or infusion.
▲ side-effects: there may be sensitivity reactions ranging from a minor rash to urticaria and joint pains, and (occasionally) to high temperature and anaphylactic shock.
✚ warning: mezlocillin should not be administered to pregnant women or to patients known to be allergic to

penicillins; it should be administered with caution to those with impaired kidney function.
Related article: BAYPEN.

MFV-Ject (*Merieux*) is the name of a series of proprietary flu VACCINES consisting of suspensions containing inactivated viral material derived from influenza viruses. It is not recommended for children.

▲ side-effects: rarely, there is local reaction together with headache and high temperature.

✚ warning: like any flu vaccine, MFV-Ject cannot control epidemics and should be used only against what seems to be the appropriate viral strain – on people who are at high risk: the elderly, patients with cardiovascular problems, and medical staff. MFV-Ject should not be administered to patients who are allergic to egg or chicken protein (in which vaccine viruses are cultured), or who are pregnant.

miconazole is an ANTIFUNGAL drug of the imidazole type, used in the treatment of many forms of fungal infection, generally by topical application (for instance, as an oral gel, as a spray powder, or as a water-miscible cream), although tablets are also available for use in oral or intestinal infection and as an injection for systemic infections. The injection contains a castor oil derivative which may cause sensitivity reactions. In solution, the drug may be used for irrigation of the bladder.

▲ side-effects: rarely, there is irritation of the skin or minor sensitivity reaction. Miconazole may cause nausea and vomiting.

✚ warning: topical treatment should be continued for more than a week after lesions or other symptoms have healed.
Related articles: DAKTARIN; DERMONISTAT.

Mictral (*Winthrop*) is a proprietary ANTIBIOTIC, available only on prescription, used primarily to treat infections of the urinary tract, including cystisis. Produced in the form of granules in a sachet for solution in water,

Mictral's major active constituents are the drug nalidixic acid and sodium citrate. It is not recommended for infants under 3 months.

▲/✚ side-effects/warning: *see* NALIDIXIC ACID.

Minims Chloramphenicol (*Smith & Nephew*) is a proprietary ANTIBIOTIC for topical application, available only on prescription, used to treat bacterial infections in the eye. Produced in the form of single-dose eye-drops, Minims Chloramphenicol is a preparation of chloramphenicol.

▲/✚ side-effects/warning: *see* CHLORAMPHENICOL.

Minims Gentamicin (*Smith & Nephew*) is a proprietary ANTIBIOTIC, available only on prescription, used to treat bacterial infections in the eye. Produced in the form of single-dose eye-drops, Minims Gentamicin is a preparation of the aminoglycoside gentamicin sulphate.

▲/✚ side-effects/warning: *see* GENTAMICIN.

Minims Neomycin (*Smith & Nephew*) is a proprietary ANTIBIOTIC, available only on prescription, used to treat bacterial infections in the eye. Produced in the form of single-dose eye-drops, it is a preparation of the aminoglycoside antibiotic neomycin.

▲/✚ side-effects/warning: *see* NEOMYCIN.

Minims Sulphacetamide Sodium (*Smith & Nephew*) is a proprietary ANTIBIOTIC, available only on prescription, used to treat local infections in the eye. Produced in the form of single-dose eye-drops, it is a preparation of the SULPHONAMIDE sulphacetamide sodium. It is no longer recommended.

▲/✚ side-effects/warning: *see* SULPHACETAMIDE.

Minocin (*Lederle*) is a proprietary broad-spectrum ANTIBIOTIC, available only on prescription, used to treat many forms of infection but particularly those of the urinary tract, the respiratory tract, skin and soft tissue (including acne), and to prevent meningococcal infections.

Produced in the form of tablets (in two strengths),
Minocin is a preparation of the TETRACYCLINE minocycline
hydrochloride. It should not be given to children aged
under 12 years or to pregnant women.
▲/✚ side-effects/warning: *see* MINOCYCLINE.

minocycline is a broad-spectrum ANTIBIOTIC, a TETRACYCLINE
with a wider range of action than other tetracyclines in
that it is effective also in treating and preventing certain
forms of meningitis. Also unlike most tetracyclines it may
be used relatively safely in a patient with impaired renal
function. Administration is oral in the form of tablets.

▲ side-effects: there may be nausea and vomiting, with
diarrhoea; dizziness and vertigo are not uncommon,
especially in female patients. Rarely, there are
sensitivity reactions.
✚ warning: minocycline should not be administered to
patients who are aged under 12 years, or who are
pregnant. It should be administered with caution to
those who are lactating or who have impaired liver or
kidney function.
Related articles: MINOCIN; TETRACYCLINES.

Mintezol (*Merck Sharp & Dohme*) is a proprietary non-
prescription ANTHELMINTIC drug, used to treat intestinal
infestations by threadworm and guinea worm, and to
assist in the treatment of resistant infections by
hookworm, whipworm and roundworm. Produced in the
form of tablets, Mintezol is a preparation of
thiabendazole.
▲/✚ side-effects/warning: *see* THIABENDAZOLE.

Miol (*Formula M1*) (Brit Cair) is a proprietary ANTISEPTIC,
available only on prescription, used in topical application
to treat inflammatory and ulcerative skin conditions.
Produced in the form of a cream and a lotion, Miol is a
preparation of various antiseptic and antifungal agents.

Miraxid (*Leo*) is a proprietary compound, orally active,
ANTIBIOTIC preparation, available only on prescription,

used to treat particularly gram-negative bacterial infections in the respiratory tract, the ear and the urinary tract. Produced in the form of tablets (in two strengths, the stronger under the name Miraxid 450, which is not recommended for children) and as a suspension for children, Miraxid is a compound preparation of the penicillins pivampicillin and pivmecillinam hydrochloride.

▲/✚ side-effects/warning: *see* PIVAMPICILLIN; PIVMECILLINAM.

M

MMR vaccine is a combined measles, mumps and rubella vaccine using live but weakened strains of the viruses (prepared in chick embryos). Health authorities are obliged to ensure that all children receive MMR vaccine before starting primary school unless there is a valid contra-indication.

▲ side-effects: as with single measles vaccine there may be fever and/or a rash about a week after; there may also be parotid gland swelling about two to three weeks after vaccination.

✚ warning: it should not be given to immunocompromised children; to children allergic to neomycin, kanamycin or egg; to children with acute febrile illness, or within three months of an immunoglobulin injection.

MMR II (*Wellcome*) is a proprietary VACCINE preparation for measles, mumps and rubella.

▲/✚ side-effects/warning: *see* MMR VACCINE.

Monaspor (*Ciba*) is a proprietary ANTIBIOTIC, available only on prescription, used to treat many forms of infection, especially those of the respiratory tract, certain bone and soft tissue infections, and those caused by the organism *Pseudomonas aeruginosa.* It is also sometimes used to ensure asepsis during surgery. Produced in the form of a powder for reconstitution as a medium for injection, Monaspor is a preparation of the CEPHALOSPORIN cefsulodin sodium.

▲/✚ side-effects/warning: *see* CEFSULODIN

Monistat (*Ortho-Cilag*) is a proprietary ANTIFUNGAL preparation for topical application, available only on prescription, used to treat yeast infections (such as thrush) of the vagina or vulva. Produced in the form of a vaginal cream and vaginal inserts (pessaries), Monistat is a preparation of miconazole nitrate. Not for use in children.
▲/✚ side-effects/warning: *see* MICONAZOLE.

monosulfiram is a parasiticidal drug used mainly in topical application to treat skin surface infestation by the itch-mite (scabies). In this it is particularly valuable in treating children. Administration is in the form of a dilute spiritous solution (generally applied topically after a hot bath).
▲ side-effects: rarely, there are sensitivity reactions.
✚ warning: keep the solution away from the eyes. During treatment, patients should avoid alcohol consumption (if absorbed, the drug may give rise to a severe reaction – as does the closely-related drug disulfiram – in the presence of alcohol).

Monotrim (*Duphar*) is a proprietary ANTIBIOTIC, available only on prescription, used to treat infections of the upper respiratory tract (particularly bronchitis and bronchial pneumonia) and of the urinary tract. Produced in the form of tablets (in two strengths), as a sugar-free suspension for dilution (the potency of the suspension once diluted is retained for 14 days), and in ampoules for injection, Monotrim is a preparation of the antibacterial drug trimethoprim. It is not recommended for children aged under 6 weeks.
▲/✚ side-effects/warning: *see* TRIMETHOPRIM.

Monphytol (*L A B*) is a proprietary non-prescription ANTIFUNGAL liquid used in topical application to treat skin infections (particularly nail) caused by fungi of the genus Tinea (such as athlete's foot). Produced in the form of a paint, Monphytol is a preparation of various acids and antibacterial agents, including salicylic acid and chlorbutol.

Moxalactam (*Lilly*) is a proprietary broad-spectrum ANTIBIOTIC, available only on prescription, used to treat many forms of bacterial infection. Produced in the form of a powder for reconstitution as a medium for injection, Moxalactam is a preparation of the CEPHALOSPORIN latamoxef disodium.

▲/✚ side-effects/warning: *see* LATAMOXEF.

Multilind (*Squibb*) is a proprietary ANTIFUNGAL preparation, available only on prescription, used in topical application to treat fungal infections, especially forms of candidiasis (such as thrush), and to relieve the symptoms of nappy rash. Produced in the form of an ointment, Multilind is a preparation of the ANTIFUNGAL agent nystatin together with zinc oxide.

▲/✚ side-effects/warning: *see* NYSTATIN.

mumps vaccine is a suspension of live but attenuated mumps viruses cultured in chick embryo tissue. It is a VACCINE not recommended for routine use in the United Kingdom, although it is readily available for patients at risk. Administration is by injection. Combined with measles and rubella vaccine it constitutes MMR vaccine.

Related article: MMR VACCINE.

Mumpsvax (*Morson*) is a proprietary MUMPS VACCINE, available only on prescription. Produced in the form of powder in a single-dose vial with diluent, Mumpsvax is a preparation of live but attenuated viruses that when injected cause the body to provide itself with antibodies against the virus. It is not recommended for children aged under 1 year.

mupirocin, or pseudomonic acid, is an ANTIBIOTIC drug, unrelated to any other antibiotic, used in topical application to treat bacterial skin infection. Administration is in the form of a water-miscible cream.

▲ side-effects: topical application may sting.

✚ warning: mupirocin should be administered with caution to patients with impaired kidney function. *Related article:* BACTROBAN.

Myambutol (*Lederle*) is a proprietary ANTITUBERCULAR drug, available only on prescription, used for the prevention and treatment of tuberculosis in conjunction with other drugs. Produced in the form of tablets (in two strengths) and as an oral powder, Myambutol is a preparation of ethambutol hydrochloride.
▲/✚ side-effects/warning: *see* ETHAMBUTOL HYDROCHLORIDE.

Myciguent (*Upjohn*) is a proprietary ANTIBIOTIC, available only on prescription, used to treat infections of the skin and the eye. Produced in the form of an ointment and an eye ointment, Myciguent is a preparation of the aminoglycoside neomycin sulphate.
▲/✚ side-effects/warning: *see* NEOMYCIN.

Mycota (*Crookes Products*) is a proprietary non-prescription ANTIFUNGAL preparation, used in topical application to treat skin infections caused by Tinea organisms (such as athlete's foot). Produced in the form of a cream, as a dusting powder, and as an aerosol spray, Mycota is a preparation of undecenoic acid and its salts.

Mynah (*Lederle*) is a proprietary ANTITUBERCULAR drug, available only on prescription, used for the prevention and treatment of tuberculosis in conjunction with other drugs. Produced in the form of tablets (in four strengths, under the names Mynah 200, Mynah 250, Mynah 300 and Mynah 365), it is a compound preparation of ethambutol hydrochloride and isoniazid. It is not recommended for children.
▲/✚ side-effects/warning: *see* ETHAMBUTOL HYDROCHLORIDE; ISONIAZID.

Mysteclin (*Squibb*) is a proprietary compound preparation with ANTIBIOTIC and ANTIFUNGAL actions, available only on prescription, used to treat infections anywhere in the body, but especially of mucous membranes. Produced in the form of capsules and as tablets, Mysteclin is a preparation of the broad-spectrum antibiotic tetracycline hydrochloride with the antifungal agent nystatin. Under the same name, a syrup is also available containing the antibiotic tetracycline and the antifungal agent amphotericin. These preparations are not recommended for children.

▲/✚ side-effects/warning: *see* AMPHOTERICIN; NYSTATIN; TETRACYCLINE.

nalidixic acid is an ANTIBIOTIC used primarily to treat gram-negative infection of the urinary tract. One of the first of the quinolone family of antibiotics, it is not active enough to achieve effective concentrations in the blood; it inhibits DNA coiling and replication in the bacterial cell. Administration is oral in the form of tablets, as a dilute suspension, or as an effervescent solution.

▲ side-effects: nausea, vomiting, diarrhoea and gastrointestinal disturbance are fairly common, but there may also be sensitivity reactions (such as urticaria or a rash). A very few patients experience visual disturbances and convulsions.

✚ warning: nalidixic acid should not be administered to patients who suffer from epilepsy, have a history of porphyria, or who are aged under 3 months. It should be administered with caution to those with kidney or liver dysfunction or who are lactating. During treatment it is advisable for patients to avoid strong sunlight.

Related articles: MICTRAL; NEGRAM; URIBEN.

Naseptin (*ICI*) is a proprietary ANTIBIOTIC preparation, available only on prescription, used to treat staphylococcal infections in and around the nostrils. Produced in the form of a cream for topical application, Naseptin is a preparation of the ANTISEPTIC chlorhexidine hydrochloride and the topical antibiotic neomycin sulphate.

▲/✚ side-effects/warning: *see* CHLORHEXIDINE; NEOMYCIN.

natamycin is an ANTIBIOTIC, an ANTIFUNGAL drug used to treat candidiasis (thrush), trichomoniasis and fungal infections of the respiratory tract. Administration is in many forms, depending on the site of infection: oral as a sugar-free suspension (sometimes in drops), topical as an aerosol inhalant and as a water-miscible cream, and also as vaginal tablets (pessaries).

✚ warning: diagnosis should preferably be confirmed (through analysis of tissue from the site of infection) before administration.

Related article: PIMAFUCIN.

Naxogin 500 (*Farmitalia Carlo Erba*) is a proprietary non-prescription ANTIPROTOZOAL, used to treat trichomonal infections of the urogenital areas. It may also be useful in the treatment of ulcerative gingivitis due to Vincent's organisms. Produced in the form of tablets, Naxogin 500 is a preparation of nimorazole. Alcohol consumption should be avoided during treatment.

▲/✚ side-effects/warning: *see* NIMORAZOLE.

Nebcin (*Lilly*) is a proprietary ANTIBIOTIC, used to treat serious infections in specific organs, such as meningitis, prostatitis, pyelonephritis and endocarditis. Produced in ampoules (in two strengths) for injection, Nebcin is a preparation of the aminoglycoside tobramycin.

▲/✚ side-effects/warning: *see* TOBRAMYCIN.

Negram (*Sterling Research*) is a proprietary ANTIBIOTIC, available only on prescription, used to treat infections of the urinary tract. Produced in the form of tablets and as a sugar-free suspension for dilution (the potency of the suspension once diluted is retained for 14 days), Negram is a preparation of the drug nalidixic acid.

▲/✚ side-effects/warning: *see* NALIDIXIC ACID.

Neo-Cortef (*Upjohn*) is a proprietary compound ANTIBIOTIC available only on prescription, used to treat bacterial infections in the outer ear and inflammation in the eye. Produced in the form of ear- or eye-drops and as an ointment, Neo-Cortef is a compound preparation of the antibiotic aminoglycoside neomycin sulphate with the CORTICOSTEROID hydrocortisone acetate.

▲/✚ side-effects/warning: *see* NEOMYCIN.

Neo-Medrone (*Upjohn*) is a proprietary CORTICOSTEROID ANTIBIOTIC preparation, available only on prescription, used for topical application to treat inflammatory skin conditions, particularly those resulting from allergy, which may be infected. Produced in the form of a cream, Neo-Medrone is a preparation of the steroid methylprednisolone acetate and the antibiotic neomycin sulphate. Neo-Medrone Lotion is also available for the treatment of acne, and additionally contains sulphur and aluminium chlorhydroxide.

▲/✚ side-effects/warning: *see* NEOMYCIN.

neomycin is a broad-spectrum ANTIBIOTIC drug of the aminoglycoside family that is effective in treating some superficial bacterial infections. Too toxic to be used in intravenous or intramuscular administration, it is nevertheless sometimes also used orally to reduce the levels of bacteria in the colon prior to intestinal surgery or examination, or in the case of liver failure. When given orally it is not absorbed from the gastrointestinal tract. Prolonged or widespread topical application may eventually lead to sensitivity reactions, and/or the development of resistance to certain strains of bacteria. Administration (most often in the form of neomycin sulphate) is oral as tablets or in solution, or topical as nose-drops, ear-drops, eye-drops, ear ointment, eye ointment or nasal spray.

▲ side-effects: prolonged use may eventually lead to temporarily impaired kidney function, malabsorption from the intestines, or to deafness. Prolonged use to treat infection in the outer ear may lead to a fungal superinfection.

✚ warning: neomycin should not be administered to patients with the neuromuscular disease myasthenia gravis, or who are pregnant. Intervals between doses should be increased for patients with impaired kidney function.

Related articles: AUDICORT; DERMOVATE-NN; DEXA-RHINASPRAY; GRANEODIN; GREGODERM; HYDRODERM; MINIMS; MYCIFRADIN; MYCIGUENT; NEO-CORTEF; NEOSPORIN; NIVEMYCIN.

Neosporin (*Calmic*) is a proprietary ANTIBIOTIC, available only on prescription, used to treat bacterial infections in the eye. Produced in the form of eye-drops, Neosporin is a compound preparation of the antibiotics

neomycin sulphate, polymyxin B sulphate and gramicidin.
▲/✚ side-effects/warning: *see* NEOMYCIN; POLYMYXIN B.

Netillin (*Kirby-Warrick*) is a proprietary form of the aminoglycoside ANTIBIOTIC netilmicin sulphate, available only on prescription. Used to treat various serious bacterial infections, it is produced in ampoules (in three · strengths) for injection.
▲/✚ side-effects/warning: *see* NETILMICIN.

netilmicin is a broad-spectrum ANTIBIOTIC, one of the aminoglycosides used (singly or in combination with other types of antibiotic) to treat serious bacterial infections caused by gram-negative bacteria, especially those that prove to be resistant to the more commonly used aminoglycoside gentamicin. Administration is by injection.
▲ side-effects: there may be temporary kidney dysfunction; any hearing deficit should be reported.
✚ warning: netilmicin should not be administered to patients with the neuromuscular disease myasthenia gravis, or who are pregnant. Intervals between doses should be increased for patients with impaired kidney functions.
Related article: NETILLIN.

niclosamide is a synthetic ANTHELMINTIC drug used to rid the body of an infestation of tapeworms. Administration is oral in the form of tablets.
▲ side-effects: there may be gastrointestinal disturbance.
✚ warning: side-effects are minimal, but in case the tapeworms are multiplying some doctors prefer to prescribe an additional anti-emetic for patients to take on waking. The dose should be administered on a relatively empty stomach, and be followed by a purgative after about 2 hours.
Related article: YOMESAN.

Nidazol (*Steinhard*) is a proprietary ANTIBIOTIC AMOEBICIDE, available only on prescription, used to treat infections by anaerobic bacteria and protozoa (particularly in the vagina) and to provide asepsis during surgery involving the large intestine or during gynaecological procedures. Produced in the form of tablets, Nidazol is a preparation of the drug metronidazole.

▲/✚ side-effects/warning: *see* METRONIDAZOLE.

nimorazole is an ANTIPROTOZOAL agent used to treat protozoal infections (such as giardiasis or trichomoniasis), particularly of the urogenital areas, and especially in cases when the major alternative drug metronidazole has failed. Administration is oral in the form of tablets.

▲ side-effects: there may be nausea and vomiting, drowsiness and vertigo; a rash may appear.

✚ warning: nimorazole should not be administered to patients with severe kidney failure or disease of the central nervous system. In cases of sexually transmitted disease, both partners should be treated even if one presents no symptoms. Alcohol consumption should be avoided during treatment. *Related article:* NAXOGIN 500.

niridazole is an ANTHELMINTIC drug used to treat infestations of guinea worms (dracontiasis). In treating guinea worm infestation the drug kills the worms and facilitates their removal from the tissues − but they do still have to be removed physically from the ulcers they cause, and the ulcers require dressing.

▲ side-effects: there may be nausea and anxiety; some patients enter a state of confusion.

✚ warning: niridazole should not be administered to patients with epilepsy; it should be administered with caution to those with impaired liver function.

nitrofurantoin is an ANTIBIOTIC that is used particularly to treat infections of the urinary tract. It is especially useful in treating kidney infections that prove to be resistant to other forms of therapy. Administration is oral in the form of tablets, as capsules, or as a suspension.

▲ side-effects: there may be loss of appetite, nausea,
vomiting and diarrhoea; impaired lung function;
peripheral neuropathy causing tingling and other
sensory disorders in the fingers and toes (patients
should report such symptoms). Rarely there is liver
damage, allergic skin reactions and blood disorders.
Urine may be coloured yellow or brown.

✚ warning: nitrofurantoin should not be administered to
patients with impaired kidney function, or who are
aged under 1 month. The drug is ineffective in
patients whose urine is alkaline. Lung, liver and
peripheral nerve function should be monitored in long-
term treatment.

Related articles: FURADANTIN; MACRODANTIN;
URANTOIN.

nitrophenol is an ANTIFUNGAL drug used in topical
application to treat skin infection (such as athlete's foot).
Administration is as an alcohol-based paint, using a
special applicator.
Related article: PHORTINEA.

Nivaquine (*May & Baker*) is a proprietary ANTIMALARIAL
drug, available only on prescription, used primarily in
combination with other drugs (such as tetracycline) for
the prevention and treatment of malaria. Some malarial
strains are now resistant to the drug. Produced in the
form of tablets, as a syrup for dilution (the potency of
the elixir once diluted is retained for 14 days), and in
ampoules for injection (during emergency treatment
only), Nivaquine is a preparation of chloroquine
sulphate.
▲/✚ side-effects/warning: *see* CHLOROQUINE.

Nivemycin (*Boots*) is a proprietary form of the
aminoglycoside ANTIBIOTIC neomycin sulphate, available
only on prescription, used to reduce bacterial levels in
the intestines before surgery. Nivemycin is produced in
the form of tablets and as an elixir.
▲/✚ side-effects/warning: *see* NEOMYCIN.

Nizoral (*Janssen*) is a proprietary ANTIFUNGAL drug, available only on prescription, used to treat both serious systemic and skin-surface fungal infections. Produced in the form of tablets, as a suspension, and as a water-miscible cream for topical application, Nizoral is a preparation of the IMIDAZOLE ketoconazole.
▲/✚ side-effects/warning: *see* KETOCONAZOLE.

Nordox (*Norton*) is a proprietary broad-spectrum ANTIBIOTIC, available only on prescription, used to treat infections of many kinds, including acne and chronic prostatitis. Produced in the form of capsules, Nordox is a preparation of the TETRACYCLINE doxycycline.
▲/✚ side-effects/warning: *see* DOXYCYCLINE.

Noxyflex (*Geistlich*) is a proprietary ANTIMICROBIAL, available only on prescription, used to treat infections of the urinary tract. Produced in the form of a powder for reconstitution as a solution for instillation into the bladder, Noxyflex is a compound preparation of the ANTIBACTERIAL/ANTIFUNGAL drug noxythiolin and the local anaesthetic amethocaine hydrochloride. A similar preparation but containing only noxythiolin is also available (under the name Noxyflex S).
▲/✚ side-effects/warning: *see* NOXYTHIOLIN.

noxythiolin is an ANTIBIOTIC that has both ANTIBACTERIAL and ANTIFUNGAL properties. A derivative of urea, its primary use is in the treatment of an infected bladder. It is introduced directly into the bladder as an irrigating solution.
✚ warning: because there may be a stinging, burning sensation on initial instillation, the drug is sometimes administered in combination with a local anaesthetic. Administration into a severely infected bladder may cause the formation of clumps of fibrous protein, which pass out with the irrigation fluid.
Related article: NOXYFLEX.

Nyspes (*DDSA Pharmaceuticals*) is a proprietary ANTIFUNGAL preparation, available only on prescription, used to treat yeast infections of the vagina or vulva. Produced in the form of vaginal inserts (pessaries), Nyspes is a preparation of nystatin.

▲/✚ side-effects/warning: *see* NYSTATIN.

Nystadermal (*Squibb*) is a proprietary CORTICOSTEROID ANTIFUNGAL cream, available only on prescription, used for topical application on areas of inflamed skin, particularly in cases of eczema that have failed to respond to less powerful drugs. Nystadermal is a preparation of the steroid triamcinolone acetonide and the antifungal nystatin.

▲/✚ side-effects/warning: *see* NYSTATIN.

Nystaform (*Bayer*) is a proprietary ANTIFUNGAL preparation, available only on prescription, used in topical application to treat fungal (particularly yeast) infections. Produced in the form of a cream and an anhydrous ointment, Nystaform is a preparation of the ANTIFUNGAL drug nystatin and one of two forms of the ANTISEPTIC chlorhexidine.

▲/✚ side-effects/warning: *see* CHLORHEXIDINE; NYSTATIN.

Nystaform-HC (*Bayer*) is a proprietary CORTICOSTEROID compound, available only on prescription, used to treat skin inflammations in which fungal and bacterial infections are suspected. Produced in the form of a water-miscible cream and an anhydrous ointment, Nystaform-HC is a preparation of the corticosteroid hydrocortisone, the ANTIFUNGAL drug nystatin, and one of two forms of the (mildly antibacterial) ANTISEPTIC chlorhexidine.

▲/✚ side-effects/warning: *see* CHLORHEXIDINE; NYSTATIN.

Nystan (*Squibb*) is the name of a proprietary group of ANTIFUNGAL preparations, available only on prescription, used to treat fungal infections (such as candidiasis, thrush). All are forms of the ANTIFUNGAL nystatin. Preparations for oral administration include tablets, a suspension, a gluten-, lactose- and sugar-free suspension, granules for reconstitution with water to form a solution,

and pastilles (for treating mouth infections). For vaginal
and vulval infections there is a vaginal cream, a gel, and
vaginal inserts (pessaries, under the name Nystavescent).
A triple pack containing tablets, gel and pessaries is
available. A water-miscible cream, gel, ointment and
dusting-powder are available for the topical treatment of
fungal skin infections.
▲/✚ side-effects/warning: *see* NYSTATIN.

nystatin is an ANTIFUNGAL drug, effective both in topical
application and when taken orally (when taken by this
method it is not absorbed and exerts its antifungal action
only in the mouth and gastrointestinal tract), primarily
used to treat the yeast infection candidiasis (thrush).
Less commonly, it is used to treat other fungal infections,
particularly in and around the mouth. Administration is
in many forms: tablets, a suspension, a solution,
pastilles, vaginal inserts (pessaries), a cream, a gel, an
ointment and a dusting-powder. It is too toxic to be
injected systemically.

▲ side-effects: treatment of the vagina may require
   additional medication to restore the natural acidity of
   the area. There may be nausea, vomiting or diarrhoea.
✚ warning: the full course of treatment must be
   completed, even if symptoms disappear earlier:
   recurrence of infection is common when treatment
   is withdrawn too hastily. Fungal infections in the
   urogenital areas imply simultaneous treatment
   of the patient's sexual partner. Treatment with
   pessaries should be continued through menstruation.
   Related articles: DERMOVATE-NN; GREGODERM; MULTILIND;
   NYSTAFORM; NYSTAN; NYSTATIN-DOME; NYSTAVESCENT;
   TINADERM-M.

Nystatin-Dome (*Bayer*) is a proprietary ANTIFUNGAL
preparation, available only on prescription, used to treat
intestinal candidiasis (thrush) and oral infections.
Produced in the form of a suspension, Nystatin-Dome is a
preparation of the ANTIFUNGAL drug nystatin.
▲/✚ side-effects/warning: *see* NYSTATIN.

Nystavescent (*Squibb*) is a proprietary ANTIFUNGAL
preparation, available only on prescription, used to treat
vaginal and vulval candidiasis (thrush). Produced in the
form of vaginal inserts (pessaries), Nystavescent is a
preparation of the ANTIFUNGAL drug nystatin.
▲/✚ side-effects/warning: *see* NYSTATIN.

Ocusol (*Boots*) is a proprietary ANTIBIOTIC preparation, available only on prescription, used to treat eye infections. Produced in the form of eye-drops, Ocusol is a preparation of the SULPHONAMIDE sulphacetamide sodium together with the astringent-cleanser zinc sulphate. It is no longer recommended.

Ophthalmadine (*SAS Pharmaceuticals*) is a proprietary preparation, available only on prescription, used to treat Herpes simplex infections of the eye. Containing a mild solution of the antiviral agent idoxuridine, it is produced in the form of eye-drops for use during the day, and eye ointment for use overnight.
▲/✚ side-effects/warning: *see* IDOXURIDINE.

Opulets (*Alcon*) is the name of a proprietary eye-drop preparation which consists of a variety of different drugs. Available only on prescription, Opulets Chloramphenicol is used to treat bacterial infections in the eye and contains the ANTIBIOTIC chloramphenicol.
▲/✚ side-effects/warning: *see* CHLORAMPHENICOL.

Oralcer (*Vitabiotics*) is a proprietary non-prescription ANTISEPTIC preparation, used to treat infections and ulcers in the mouth. Produced in the form of lozenges, Oralcer contains clioquinol and ascorbic acid (vitamin C).
▲/✚ side-effects/warning: *see* CLIOQUINOL.

Oraldene (*Warner-Lambert*) is a proprietary non-prescription ANTISEPTIC preparation, used to treat sores and ulcers in the mouth. Produced in the form of a mouth-wash, Oraldene's active constituent is hexetidine.

Orbenin (*Beecham*) is a proprietary ANTIBIOTIC, available only on prescription, used to treat bacterial infections, and especially staphylococcal infections that prove to be resistant to penicillin. Produced in the form of capsules (in two strengths), as a syrup for dilution, and as powder for reconstitution as injections, Orbenin's active constituent is cloxacillin.
▲/✚ side-effects/warning: *see* CLOXACILLIN.

Otosporin (*Calmic*) is a proprietary ANTIBIOTIC preparation, available only on prescription, used to treat infections and inflammation in the outer ear. Produced in the form of ear-drops, Otosporin contains the CORTICOSTEROID hydrocortisone and the ANTIBIOTICS neomycin sulphate and polymyxin B sulphate.

✚ warning: *see* CORTICOSTEROIDS; NEOMYCIN SULPHATE; POLYMYXIN B SULPHATE.

O

oxamniquine is an ANTHELMINTIC drug that is effective in treating the form of bilharzia (schistosomiasis) caused by the intestinal blood vessel parasite *Schistosoma mansoni*, not uncommon in Africa, the West Indies, and South and Central America. Administration is oral, and toxicity is minimal.

Oxymycin (*DDSA Pharmaceuticals*) is a proprietary ANTIBIOTIC, available only on prescription, used to treat many microbial infections, such as severe acne vulgaris and exacerbations of chronic bronchitis. Produced in the form of tablets, Oxymycin's active constituent is the tetracycline oxytetracycline dihydrate.

✚ warning: *see* OXYTETRACYCLINE.

oxytetracycline is a broad-spectrum ANTIBIOTIC, one of the TETRACYCLINES, used to treat many serious infections, particularly those of the urogenital organs and skin or mucous membrane, of the bones, and of the respiratory passages. It may also be used to treat acne, although it is not suitable for children aged under 12 years. Administration is oral in the form of tablets or syrup.

▲ side-effects: there may be nausea and vomiting, with diarrhoea; hypersensitivity reactions may occur, as may photosensitivity (sensitivity of the skin and eyes to light), but both are rare.

✚ warning: oxytetracycline should not be administered to patients who are pregnant, or who have kidney failure. It should be administered with caution to patients who are lactating. Some bacterial strains have now become resistant to the drug.

Related articles: BERKMYCEN; GALENOMYCIN; IMPERACIN; OXYMYCIN; TERRAMYCIN; tetracyclines; UNIMYCIN.

Paludrine (*ICI*) is a proprietary non-prescription drug used in the prevention of malaria (*see* ANTIMALARIAL). Produced in the form of tablets, Paludrine is a preparation of proguanil hydrochloride.
▲/✚ side-effects/warning: *see* PROGUANIL.

Panmycin (*Upjohn*) is a proprietary ANTIBIOTIC available only on prescription, used to treat many forms of infection. Produced in the form of capsules or syrup, Panmycin is a preparation of the broad-spectrum antibiotic tetracycline hydrochloride. It is not recommended for use in children.
▲/✚ side-effects/warning: *see* TETRACYCLINE.

*pediculicidal drugs kill lice of the genus Pediculus, which infest either the body or the scalp − or both − and cause intense itching. Scratching tends only to damage the skin surface, and may eventually cause weeping lesions or bacterial infection as well. Best known and most used pediculicides include malathion and carbaryl; the once commonly used lindane is now no longer recommended for lice on the scalp because resistant strains of lice have emerged. Administration is topical, generally in the form of a lotion; contact between drug and skin should be as long as possible (at least two hours), which is why shampoos are less commonly used.
▲/✚ side-effects/warning: *see* BENZYL BENZOATE; CARBARYL; LINDANE; MALATHION.

Penbritin (*Beecham*) is a proprietary form of the broad-spectrum penicillin ampicillin, available only on prescription. An ANTIBIOTIC used mainly to treat infections of the respiratory passages, the middle ear and the urinary tract, it is also effective against gonorrhoea. Penbritin is produced in the form of capsules (in two strengths), as tablets for children, as a syrup (in two strengths, for dilution; the potency of the syrup once diluted is retained for 7 days), as a children's suspension for use with a pipette, and as powder for reconstitution as a solution for injections.
▲/✚ side-effects/warning: *see* AMPICILLIN.

penicillin G is a term for the ANTIBIOTIC more commonly known as benzylpenicillin.
see BENZYLPENICILLIN.

penicillin V is a term for the ANTIBIOTIC more commonly known as phenoxymethylpenicillin.
see PHENOXYMETHYLPENICILLIN.

penicillin VK is a term for the potassium salt of the ANTIBIOTIC more commonly known as phenoxymethylpenicillin.
see PHENOXYMETHYLPENICILLIN.

penicillinases are enzymes, produced by some bacteria, that inhibit or completely neutralize the antibacterial activity of many forms of PENICILLIN. Treatment of infections caused by bacteria that produce penicillinases has generally therefore to be undertaken either with penicillinase-resistant penicillins, such as flucloxacillin, or with other types of antibiotic. Therapeutically, however, penicillinases can be used (in purified form) to treat sensitivity reactions to penicillin, or in tests to identify micro-organisms in blood samples taken from patients who are taking penicillin.

penicillins are ANTIBIOTIC drugs that work by interfering with the synthesis of bacterial cell walls. The early penicillins were effective against principally gram-positive bacteria but also the gram-negative organisms (Neisseria) causing gonorrheoa and meningitis, as well as the organism causing syphilis. Later penicillins, e.g. ampicillin and pipercillin, expanded the spectrum to a much wider range of gram-negative organisms. They are absorbed rapidly by most (but not all) body tissues and fluids, perfuse through the kidneys, and are excreted in the urine. One great disadvantage of penicillins is that many patients are allergic to them − allergy to one means allergy to them all − and may have reactions that range from a minor rash right up to anaphylactic shock, which may be fatal. Otherwise they are remarkably non-

P

toxic. Very high dosage may rarely cause convulsions, haemolytic anaemia, or abnormally high body levels of sodium or potassium, with consequent symptoms. Best known and most used penicillins include benzylpenicillin (penicillin G, the first of the penicillins), phenoxymethylpenicillin (penicillin V), flucloxacillin, ampicillin and amoxycillin. Those taken orally tend to cause diarrhoea; and there is a risk with broad-spectrum penicillins of allowing a superinfection to develop.

▲/✚ side-effects/warning: *see* AMOXYCILLIN; AMPICILLIN; AZLOCILLIN; BACAMPICILLIN HYDROCHLORIDE; BENETHAMINE PENICILLIN; BENZATHINE PENICILLIN; BENZYLPENICILLIN; CARBENICILLIN; CARFECILLIN SODIUM; CICLACILLIN; CLOXACILLIN; FLUCLOXACILLIN; MECILLINAM; METHICILLIN SODIUM; MEZLOCILLIN; PHENETHICILLIN; PHENOXYMETHYLPENICILLIN; PIPERACILLIN; PIVAMPICILLIN; PIVMECILLINAM; PROCAINE PENICILLIN; TALAMPICILLIN HYDROCHLORIDE; TICARCILLIN.

Penidural (*Wyeth*) is a proprietary ANTIBIOTIC, available only on prescription, used to treat many forms of infection (including syphilis) and to prevent fresh episodes of rheumatic fever following from a streptococcal sore throat/tonsillitis. Produced in the form of a suspension for dilution (the potency of the suspension once diluted is retained for 14 days), as drops for children, and in vials for injection (under the name Penidural-LA), Penidural is a preparation of benzathine penicillin.

▲/✚ side-effects/warning: *see* BENZATHINE PENICILLIN.

pentamidine is an ANTI-PROTOZOAL drug that is used to treat pneumonia caused by the protozoan micro-organism *Pneumocystis carinii* in patients whose immune system has been suppressed (either following transplant surgery or because of a condition such as AIDS). However, it is not ordinarily available in the United Kingdom. It is administered either by injection or inhalation. Both methods of administration can cause acute episodes of low blood pressure.

Pentostam (*Wellcome*) is a proprietary ANTIPROTOZOAL preparation of the drug sodium stibogluconate (an organic compound of antimony), available only on prescription, used to treat skin infections by protozoal micro-organisms of the genus *Leishmania* (leishmaniasis). It is produced in a solution for injection.

▲/✚ side-effects/warning: *see* SODIUM STIBOGLUCONATE.

pertussis vaccine, or whooping cough VACCINE, is a suspension of dead pertussis bacteria (*Bordetella pertussis*) that is injected to cause the body's own defence mechanisms to form antibodies and thus provide immunity. It is available on prescription by itself, but it is most commonly administered as one element in the triple vaccination procedure involving diphtheria-pertussis-tetanus (DPT) vaccine. The vaccine remains the subject of some controversy over the number of children who may or may not have been brain-damaged by inoculation. It would in any case be extremely difficult to attribute such damage definitively to the use of the vaccine, and law suits brought to court have had to rely on solely statistical evidence of probability or possibility. However, the statistics do not make for comfortable reading by parents: in the 1980s it was estimated that permanent brain damage might be expected to occur in 1 in 300,000 vaccinations. Obviously, people would prefer to have no risk whatever, but sometimes disregard the fact that the likelihood of catching whooping cough and developing serious neurological complications is statistically greater. Administration is by three injections one month apart.

▲ side-effects: there may be a local reaction of swelling and inflammation around the injection site. Very rarely there is a generalized reaction within 48 hours, with fever being a prominent symptom.

✚ warning: in general, pertussis vaccine should not be administered to children who suffer a severe local or general reaction to the initial dose, or who have a history of brain damage at birth or of cerebral irritation or seizures. It should be administered with

extreme caution to children whose relatives have a
history of seizures or who appear to have any form of
neurological disorder.

see also DIPHTHERIA-PERTUSSIS-TETANUS (DPT) VACCINE.

Pevaryl (*Ortho-Cilag*) is a proprietary non-prescription
ANTIFUNGAL drug, used in topical application to treat
fungal infections on the skin such as nail infections, and
in the genital areas. Produced in the form of a cream, a
lotion and a spray-powder in an aerosol unit, Pevaryl is a
preparation of econazole nitrate.

▲/✚ side-effects/warning: ECONAZOLE NITRATE.

phenethicillin is a penicillin-type ANTIBIOTIC that is used
both to treat bacterial infection and to prevent it. It has a
similar spectrum of activity and usage to
phenoxymethylpenicillin. Administration (as a potassium
salt) is oral in the form of capsules or a dilute syrup.

▲ side-effects: there may be sensitivity reactions ranging
from a minor rash to urticaria and joint pains,
diarrhoea and (occasionally) to high temperature or
anaphylactic shock.

✚ warning: phenethicillin should not be administered to
patients who are known to be allergic to penicillins; it
should be administered with caution to those with
impaired kidney function.

Related article: BROXIL.

phenoxymethylpenicillin, or penicillin V, is a widely-
used ANTIBIOTIC, particularly effective in treating
tonsillitis, infection of the middle ear, and some skin
infections, and to prevent recurrent streptococcal throat
infection which can lead to episodes of rheumatic fever.
Administration (as a potassium salt sometimes called
phenoxymethylpenicillin VK) is oral in the form of
tablets or liquids.

▲ side-effects: there may be sensitivity reactions ranging
from a minor rash to urticaria and joint pains, and
(occasionally) to high temperature or anaphylactic
shock.

✚ warning: phenoxymethylpenicillin should not be administered to patients known to be allergic to penicillins; it should be administered with caution to those with impaired kidney function.
Related articles: APSIN VK; CRYSTAPEN V; DISTAQUAINE V-K; ECONOCIL VK; STABILLIN V-K; V-CIT-K.

Phytex (*Pharmax*) is a proprietary non-prescription ANTIFUNGAL drug, used to treat fungal infections in the skin and nails. Produced in the form of a paint for topical application, Phytex is a preparation of various natural acids, including salicylic acid, together with methyl salicylate.
▲/✚ side-effects/warning: Hypersensitivity reactions may occur.

Phytocil (*Radiol*) is a proprietary non-prescription ANTIFUNGAL drug, used in topical application, to treat skin infections, especially athlete's foot. Produced in the form of a cream, and a powder in a sprinkler tin, Phytocil is a compound preparation that includes several minor antifungal constituents, including salicylic acid.
▲/✚ side-effects/warning: Hypersensitivity may occur.

Pimafucin (*Brocades*) is a proprietary ANTIFUNGAL drug, available only on prescription, used to treat fungal infections (such as candidiasis), particularly in the mouth, respiratory tract and vagina. Produced in the form of a sugar-free oral suspension, a suspension for inhalation, as vaginal inserts (pessaries) and as vaginal cream, and as a water-miscible cream for topical application to the skin, Pimafucin is a preparation of natamycin.
▲/✚ side-effects/warning: *see* NATAMYCIN.

piperacillin is a broad-spectrum penicillin-type ANTIBIOTIC closely related to ampicillin, used to treat many serious or compound forms of bacterial infection, particularly those caused by *Pseudomonas aeruginosa*.
Administration is by injection or infusion.

P

▲ side-effects: there may be sensitivity reactions ranging from a minor rash to urticaria and joint pains, and (occasionally) to high temperature or anaphylactic shock.

✚ warning: piperacillin should not be administered to patients known to be allergic to penicillins; it should be administered with caution to those with impaired kidney function.

Related article: Pipril.

piperazine is an ANTHELMINTIC drug, one of the phenothiazine derivatives, used to treat infestation by roundworms or threadworms. Treatment should take no longer than seven days; in the treatment of some species a single dose is sufficient. Administration (as piperazine citrate, piperazine hydrate or piperazine phosphate) is oral in the form of tablets, a syrup or a dilute elixir.

▲ side-effects: there may be nausea and vomiting, with diarrhoea; there may also be urticaria. Rarely, there is dizziness and lack of muscular co-ordination.

✚ warning: piperazine should not be administered to patients with liver disease or epilepsy; it should be administered with caution to those with impaired kidney function, neurological disease or psychiatric disorders.

Related articles: Antepar; Ascalix; Pripsen.

Pipril (*Lederle*) is a proprietary broad-spectrum penicillin-type ANTIBIOTIC, available only on prescription, used to treat many serious or compound forms of bacterial infection, particularly those caused by *Pseudomonas aeruginosa*. Produced in the form of a powder in vials (in two strengths) and in an infusion bottle, Pipril is a preparation of piperacillin.

▲/✚ side-effects/warning: *see* PIPERACILLIN.

pivampicillin is a more readily absorbed form of the ANTIBIOTIC ampicillin that is converted in the body to ampicillin after absorption. It has similar actions and uses.

▲/✚ side-effects/warning: *see* AMPICILLIN.

Related articles: Miraxid; Pondocillin.

pivmecillinam hydrochloride is a form of the ANTIBIOTIC mecillinam that can be taken orally. It has similar actions and uses.

▲/✚ side-effects/warning: *see* MECILLINAM.

    Related articles: MIRAXID; SELEXID.

pneumococcal vaccine is a VACCINE against pneumonia, consisting a suspension of polysaccharides from a number of capsular types of pneumococci, administered by subcutaneous or intramuscular injection. Like the influenza vaccine, it is intended really only for those people at risk from infection in a community — and at risk from an identified pneumococcal strain prevalent within that community. Immunity is reckoned to last for about 5 years.

✚ warning: vaccination should not be given to patients who are aged under 2 years, who have any form of infection, or who are pregnant. It should be administered with caution to those with cardiovascular or respiratory disease. Some patients experience sensitivity reactions, which may be serious. Although protection may last for only 5 years, revaccination should be avoided because of the risk of adverse reactions.

Pneumovax (*Morson*) is a proprietary form of the pneumococcal vaccine, available only on prescription for the immunization of personnel for whom the risk of contracting pneumococcal pneumonia is unusually high.

✚ warning: see PNEUMOCOCCAL VACCINE.

poliomyelitis vaccine is a VACCINE available in two types. Poliomyelitis vaccine, inactivated, is a suspension of dead viruses injected into the body for the body to generate antibodies and so become immune. Poliomyelitis vaccine live, is a suspension of live but attenuated polio viruses (of polio virus types 1, 2 and 3) for oral administration. In the United Kingdom, the live vaccine is the medium of choice, and the administration is generally simultaneous with the administration of the diphtheria-

P

pertussis-tetanus (DPT) vaccine − three times during the first year of life, and a booster at school entry age. The inactivated vaccine remains available for those patients for whom there are contra-indications.

✚ warning: poliomyelitis vaccine should not be administered to patients known to have immunodeficiency disorders, who have diarrhoea or cancer, where there is infection, or who are pregnant. Parents of a recently inoculated baby must take extra hygienic precautions when changing its nappies.

pol/vac (inact) is an abbreviation for poliomyelitis vaccine, inactivated.
see POLIOMYELITIS VACCINE.

pol/vac (oral) is an abbreviation for poliomyelitis vaccine, live (oral).
see POLIOMYELITIS VACCINE.

Polybactrin (*Calmic*) is a proprietary ANTIBIOTIC, available only on prescription, used either as a powder for reconstitution as a solution for bladder irrigation to treat bladder and urethral infections, or in the form of a powder spray as a topical treatment for minor burns and wounds. In each case, active constituents are polymyxin B sulphate, neomycin sulphate and bacitracin.

Polyfax (*Calmic*) is a proprietary ANTIBIOTIC preparation, available only on prescription, used by topical application to treat infections of the skin and the eye. Produced in the form of an ointment in a paraffin base, and as an eye ointment, Polyfax is a preparation of polymyxin B sulphate and bacitracin zinc.

▲/✚ side-effects/warning: *see* POLYMYXIN B.

polymyxin B is an ANTIBIOTIC used to treat several forms of bacterial infection, particularly those of the gram-negative organisms, including *Pseudomonas aeruginosa*. Its use would be more popular were it not so toxic. Because of its toxicity, administration (as polymyxin B sulphate) is usually topical in the form of solutions (as in eye-drops and ear-drops) or ointments, and only rarely by injection or infusion.

▲ side-effects: there may be numbness and tingling in the limbs, blood and protein in the urine, dizziness, breathlessness and overall weakness.

✚ warning: polymyxin B should not be administered to patients with the neuromuscular disease myasthenia gravis; it should be administered with caution to those with impaired kidney function.

Related articles: AEROSPORIN; GREGODERM; NEOSPORIN; OTOSPORIN; OTOTRIPS; POLYBACTRIN; POLYFAX; POLYTRIM; TRIBIOTIC.

polynoxylin is a mild ANTIFUNGAL agent. It is used primarily to treat fungal infections of the mouth and throat (such as thrush). Administration is oral in the form of lozenges.

Related article: ANAFLEX.

Polytrim (*Wellcome*) is a proprietary ANTIBIOTIC, available only on prescription, used in the form of eye-drops to treat bacterial infections in the eye. Polytrim is a preparation of the antibiotics trimethoprim and polymyxin B sulphate.

▲/✚ side-effects/warning: *see* POLYMYXIN B; TRIMETHOPRIM.

Pondocillin (*Burgess*) is a proprietary ANTIBIOTIC, available only on prescription, used to treat systemic bacterial infections and infections of the upper respiratory tract, of the ear, nose and throat, and of the urogenital tracts. Produced in the form of tablets, as a sugar-free suspension, and as granules in sachets, Pondocillin is a preparation of the broad-spectrum penicillin pivampicillin.

▲/✚ side-effects/warning: *see* PIVAMPICILLIN.

potassium permanganate is a general DISINFECTANT used in solution for cleaning burns and abrasions and maintaining asepsis in wounds that are suppurating or weeping.

✚warning: avoid splashing mucous membranes, to which it is an irritant. It also stains skin and fabric.

povidone-iodine is a complex of iodine on an organic carrier, used as an ANTISEPTIC in topical application to the skin, especially in sensitive areas (such as the vulva), and as a mouth wash. Produced in the form of a gel, a solution, or vaginal inserts (pessaries), it works by slowly releasing the iodine it contains.

▲side-effects: rarely, there may be sensitivity reactions.

✚warning: povidone-iodine should not be used during pregnancy or while lactating.
Related articles: BETADINE; DISADINE DP; VIDENE.

praziquantel is an ANTHELMINTIC, the drug of first choice in treating infections caused by schistosomes, the worms that can colonize the veins of a human host and cause bilharziasis. It is effective against all three human schistosomes. It is also useful in the treatment of tapeworm infestations. Praziquantel is of low toxicity and is active when taken orally. The drug is not marketed in the United Kingdom.

primaquine is an ANTIMALARIAL drug used to destroy parasitic forms in the liver which are not destroyed by chloroquine. It is given for two to three weeks following successful killing by chloroquine of all blood cell forms of the malarial parasite. Administration is oral in the form of tablets.

▲side-effects: there may be nausea and vomiting, anorexia and jaundice. Rarely, there are blood disorders or depression of the bone-marrow's capacity for forming new blood cells.

✚warning: a blood count is essential before administration to check that a patient has sufficient blood levels of a specific enzyme, without which the presence of the drug may cause blood disorders. Primaquine should be administered with caution to patients who are pregnant.

Prioderm (*Napp*) is a proprietary non-prescription drug used to treat infestations of the scalp and pubic hair by lice (pediculosis), or of the skin by the itch-mite (scabies). Produced in the form of a lotion in an alcohol base, and as a cream shampoo, Prioderm is a preparation of the insecticide malathion.

▲/✚ side-effects/warning: *see* MALATHION.

Pripsen (*Reckitt & Colman*) is a proprietary non-prescription ANTHELMINTIC, used to treat infections by threadworm and roundworm. Produced in the form of an oral powder, Pripsen is a preparation of the phenothiazine derivative piperazine phosphate with various stimulant laxatives, and is not recommended for children aged under 3 months.

▲/✚ side-effects/warning: *see* PIPERAZINE.

probenecid is a drug that can be used to inhibit the excretion by the kidneys of penicillin and cephalosporin antibiotics, thus prolonging the antibiotics' effects.

▲ side-effects: side-effects are uncommon, but there may be nausea and vomiting, headache and flushing, dizziness and a rash, and frequent urination. Some patients experience blood disorders.

✚ warning: probenecid should not be administered to patients with blood disorders or kidney stones, who are undergoing an acute attack of gout, or who are already taking salicylate drugs (such as aspirin). It should be administered with caution to patients with peptic ulcer. The drug is ineffective in a patient with impaired kidney function. Initial administration should be accompanied by the administration of colchicine to ward off acute gout attacks. Adequate fluid intake is essential.

procaine penicillin is a penicillin-type ANTIBIOTIC that is essentially a rather insoluble salt of benzylpenicillin. It is primarily used in long-lasting intramuscular (depot) injections to treat conditions such as syphilis and gonorrhoea, but may also be used to treat the equally

P

serious condition gas gangrene following amputation. Benzylpenicillin is released slowly into the blood over a period of days, thus avoiding the need for frequent injections. Administration is by intramuscular injection.

▲/✚ side-effects/warning: *see* BENZYLPENICILLIN.

proguanil is an ANTIMALARIAL drug used to try to prevent the contraction of malaria by travellers in tropical countries. Its effectiveness is not guaranteed, and the traveller is advised to take measures as far as possible to avoid being bitten by mosquitoes. In some areas concurrent prophylactic treatment with chloroquine is advised. Administration (as proguanil hydrochloride) is oral in the form of tablets.

▲ side-effects: there may be mild gastric disorder.

✚ warning: proguanil should be administered with caution to patients who suffer from impaired kidney function.
Related article: PALUDRINE.

prothionamide is an ANTITUBERCULAR drug also used to treat leprosy. It is not marketed in the United Kingdom.

Pyopen (*Beecham*) is a proprietary ANTIBIOTIC, available only on prescription, used mainly to treat infections of the urinary tract and upper respiratory tract, and septicaemia. Produced in the form of a powder for reconstitution as a medium for injection, Pyopen is a preparation of the PENICILLIN carbenicillin.

▲/✚ side-effects/warning: *see* CARBENICILLIN.

pyrantel is a broad-spectrum ANTHELMINTIC drug used in the treatment of infections by roundworm, threadworm, hookworm and whipworm. Administration is oral in the form of tablets.

▲ side-effects: pyrantel rarely has side-effects, but it may occasionally produce mild nausea.

✚ warning: pyrantel should not be administered to patients with liver disease, or to children aged under 6 months.
Related article: COMBANTRIN.

pyrazinamide is an ANTIBACTERIAL that is one of the major
forms of treatment for tuberculosis, and particularly
tuberculous meningitis. It is used generally in
combination (to cover resistance and for maximum effect)
with other drugs such as isoniazid and rifampicin.
Treatment lasts for between 6 and 9 months, depending
on the severity of the condition and on the specific drug
combination. Because pyrazinamide is active only
against dividing forms of *Mycobacterium tuberculosis* it is
most effective in the early stages of treatment, i.e. the
first few months. Administration is oral in the form of
tablets.

▲ side-effects: there may be symptoms of liver
malfunction, including high temperature, severe
weight loss and jaundice. There may be nausea and
vomiting, sensitivity reactions such as urticaria,
and/or blood disorders.

✚ warning: pyrazinamide should not be administered to
patients with liver disease; it should be administered
with caution to patients with impaired liver function,
porphyria, diabetes or gout. Regular checks on liver
function are essential.

Related article: ZINAMIDE.

pyrimethamine is an ANTIMALARIAL drug used primarily to
prevent contraction of malaria by travellers in tropical
countries. However, if the disease is contracted, the drug
is effective in treating forms of malaria that are resistant
to treatment with the more commonly-prescribed drug
chloroquine, and additionally prevents most relapses of
benign tertiary forms. Pyrimethamine can also be used,
along with a sulphonamide, to treat the protozoal
infection toxoplasmosis. Administration is oral in the
form of tablets.

▲ side-effects: suppression of the bone-marrow's capacity
for forming new blood cells occurs with prolonged
treatment. There may be rashes.

✚ warning: pyrimethamine should be administered with
caution to patients with impaired liver or kidney

function, or who are taking folic acid supplements (for example, during pregnancy). High doses require regular blood counts.
Related articles: DARAPRIM; FANSIDAR; MALOPRIM.

Quellada (*Stafford-Miller*) is a proprietary non-prescription preparation of the antiparasitic lindane, used to treat infestation of the skin of the trunk and limbs by itch-mites (scabies) or by lice (pediculosis). It is also used to treat hair lice infestations. Produced in the form of a lotion, it is also available as a shampoo (under the name Quellada Application PC). Neither is recommended for children aged under 1 month. Children under 6 months should be treated only under medical supervision. Both are for external use only.

▲/✚ side-effects/warning: *see* LINDANE.

quinine is an alkaloid of cinchona which was for years used as the main treatment for malaria. Now synthetic and less toxic drugs — such as chloroquine and proguanil — have replaced it almost entirely, although it is still used (in the form of quinine sulphate or quinine hydrochloride) in cases that prove to be resistant to the newer drugs or for emergency cases in which large doses are necessary. Administration is oral in the form of tablets, or by infusion.

▲ side-effects: toxic effects — corporately called cinchonism — include nausea, headache and abdominal pain, visual disturbances, ringing in the ears (tinnitus), a rash and confusion. Some patients may experience visual disturbances and temporary blindness, others may undergo further sensitivity reactions.

✚ warning: quinine should not be administered to patients who suffer from inflammation of the optic nerves or any condition that produces blood in the urine; it should be administered with caution to those who suffer from heart block or atrial fibrillation ("palpitations"), or who are pregnant.

Quinoped (*Quinoderm*) is a proprietary non-prescription topical ANTIFUNGAL preparation for the treatment of skin infections such as athlete's foot. Produced in the form of a cream in an astringent base, Quinoped is a compound of the keratolytic benzoyl peroxide and the antifungal, antibacterial and deodorant potassium hydroxyquinoline sulphate.

Q

rabies vaccine is specifically a VACCINE and not a treatment for rabies, administered to medical workers and relatives who may come into contact with hydrophobic patients or to patients who have been bitten by an animal that might or might not be rabid. It should be routinely administered to people who work with animals (e.g. vets) to prevent rabies. The vaccine is of a type known as a human diploid cell vaccine and has no known contra-indications. It is freeze-dried and produced in vials with a diluent for injection. The timing of injections within courses of injections depends on whether treatment is simply preventative (in which case the regime is usually two doses over 1 month and a third dose after 6-12 months, and possibly a booster every 3 years, depending on the risk of infection), or if rabies in a patient is suspected or confirmed (in which case medical workers and their relatives are injected on days 0, 3, 7, 14, 30 and 90 after exposure).

Retcin (*DDSA Pharmaceuticals*) is a proprietary ANTIBIOTIC, available only on prescription, used to treat many infections (including serious infections such as legionnaires' disease and inflammation of the prostate gland) and to prevent others (such as diphtheria or whooping cough), especially in patients who are allergic to penicillin-type antibiotics. Produced in the form of tablets, Retcin is a preparation of erythromycin.
▲/✚ side-effects/warning: *see* ERYTHROMYCIN.

Rifadin (*Merrell*) is a proprietary ANTITUBERCULAR drug, available only on prescription, generally used in combination with other antitubercular drugs. It may also be used to treat leprosy in dapsone-resistant cases. Produced in the form of capsules (in two strengths), as a syrup, and in the form of a powder for reconstitution as a medium for intravenous infusion, Rifadin is a preparation of the ANTIBIOTIC rifampicin.
▲/✚ side-effects/warning: *see* RIFAMPICIN.

rifampicin is an ANTIBIOTIC that is one of the principal drugs used in the treatment of tuberculosis. Even so, it is used generally in combination (to cover resistance and for maximum effect) with other antitubercular drugs such as isoniazid or streptomycin. Treatment lasts for between 6 and 9 months depending on severity and on the specific drug combination, but the use of rifampicin tends to imply the shorter duration. The drug inhibits *Mycobacterium tuberculosis* and sensitive gram-positive bacteria by inhibiting the bacterial RNA polymerase enzyme. Rifampicin is also effective in the treatment of leprosy in cases where the usual antileprotic drug dapsone has failed. Administration is oral in the form of capsules, tablets or a syrup, or by injection or infusion.

▲ side-effects: there are often gastrointestinal problems involving nausea, vomiting, diarrhoea and weight loss; many patients also undergo the symptoms of flu, which may also lead to breathlessness. Rarely, there is kidney failure, liver dysfunction, jaundice, alteration in the composition of the blood and/or discoloration of the urine, saliva and other body secretions. Sensitivity reactions, such as a rash or urticaria, can occur.

✚ warning: rifampicin should not be administered to patients with jaundice; it should be administered with caution to those with impaired liver function, who are alcoholic, or who are pregnant or lactating. One other effect of the drug is that soft contact lenses may become discoloured.

Rifampicin causes the induction of liver enzymes which are responsible for metabolizing many other drugs; these other drugs therefore may be less effective than usual, e.g. oral contraceptives are metabolized more rapidly, and at the usual dose they will not provide safe contraception.

Related articles: RIFADIN; RIFATER; RIFINAH; RIMACTANE; RIMACTAZID.

Rifater (*Merrell*) is a proprietary ANTITUBERCULAR drug, available only on prescription, used to treat pulmonary tuberculosis in the initial intensive phase. Produced in the form of tablets, Rifater is a combined preparation of rifampicin, isoniazid and pyrazinamide. It is not recommended for children.

▲/✚ side-effects/warning: *see* ISONIAZID; PYRAZINAMIDE; RIFAMPICIN.

Rifinah (*Merrell*) is a proprietary ANTITUBERCULAR drug, available only on prescription, used to treat tuberculosis. Produced in the form of tablets (in two strengths, under the trade names Rifinah 150 and Rifinah 300), Rifinah is a combined preparation of rifampicin and isoniazid.

▲/✚ side-effects/warning: *see* ISONIAZID; RIFAMPICIN.

Rimactane (*Ciba*) is a proprietary ANTITUBERCULAR drug, available only on prescription, used in combination with other antitubercular drugs. Produced in the form of capsules (in two strengths), as a syrup and in the form of a powder for reconstitution as a medium for intravenous infusion, Rimactane is a preparation of the ANTIBIOTIC rifampicin.

▲/✚ side-effects/warning: *see* RIFAMPICIN.

Rimactazid (*Ciba*) is a proprietary ANTITUBERCULAR drug, available only on prescription, used singly or in combination with other antitubercular drugs. It may also be used to treat certain other bacterial infections. Produced in the form of tablets (in two strengths, under the names Rimactazid 150 and Rimactazid 300), Rimactazid is a combined preparation of the ANTIBIOTICS rifampicin and isoniazid.

▲/✚ side-effects/warning: *see* ISONIAZID; RIFAMPICIN.

Rimevax (*Smith, Kline & French*) is a proprietary VACCINE against measles (rubeola), available only on prescription. It is a powdered preparation of live but attenuated measles viruses for administration with a diluent by injection to provide active immunization. Rimevax is not recommended for administration to children aged under 12 months.

▲ side-effects: there may be inflammation at the site of injection. Rarely, there may be high temperature, headache, a rash, swelling of the lymph glands, pain in the joints and/or a cough. Very rarely, there are allergic reactions, and in a few patients convulsions have followed the high fever.

✚ warning: Rimevax should not be administered to patients with any infection, particularly tuberculosis and other infections of the airways; who are allergic to eggs (the viruses are cultured in chick-embryo tissue); who have known immune-system abnormalities, including leukemia; who are known to be allergic to neomycin; who are pregnant; or who are already taking corticosteroid drugs, cytotoxic drugs or undergoing radiation treatment. It should be administered with caution to those with epilepsy (especially children) or any other condition potentially involving convulsive fits, and those who have recently had a blood transfusion.

Rimifon (*Roche*) is a proprietary ANTITUBERCULAR drug, available only on prescription, used in combination with other antitubercular drugs. Produced in ampoules for injection, Rimifon is a preparation of the ANTIBIOTIC isoniazid.

▲/✚ side-effects/warning: *see* ISONIAZID.

Roccal (*Winthrop*) is a proprietary non-prescription DISINFECTANT, used to cleanse the skin before operations, to cleanse wounds, to sterilize dressings, to cleanse breast and nipple shields, and also as a vaginal douche. Produced in the form of a solution, Roccal is a preparation of benzalkonium chloride. A concentrated form is available (under the name Roccal Concentrate 10X) for the preparation of the same solution, using purified water. Roccal should not be used with soap.

rosaxacin is another name for the antibacterial agent acrosoxacin.
see ACROSOXACIN.

Rotersept (*Roterpharma*) is a proprietary non-prescription DISINFECTANT, used to treat sore and cracked nipples before and after breast-feeding. Produced in the form of spray in an aerosol, Rotersept is a preparation of chlorhexidine gluconate.

▲/✚ side-effects/warning: *see* CHLORHEXIDINE.

rubella vaccine is a VACCINE against German measles (rubella) that is medically recommended for pre-pubertal girls between the ages of 10 and 14, and for medical staff who as potential carriers might put pregnant women at risk from infection, and also for women of child-bearing age, because German measles during pregnancy constitutes a serious risk to the foetus. As a precaution vaccination should not take place if the patient is pregnant or likely to become pregnant within the following 3 months. The vaccine is prepared as a freeze-dried suspension of live but attenuated viruses grown in cell cultures; administration is by injection.

Related articles: ALMEVAX; ERVEVAX; MERUVAX II.

rub/vac is an abbreviation for rubella vaccine.
see RUBELLA VACCINE.

salicylic acid is an ANTIFUNGAL drug that is used to treat minor skin infections such as athlete's foot.
Administration is topical, in the form of a solution, a collodion (paint or gel), as an ointment − or, in combination with precipitated sulphur, as an ointment or a cream − as a shampoo, and even in an impregnated adhesive plaster.

▲ side-effects: side-effects are rare, confined largely to the effects of too widescale an application (*see below*) and to sensitivity reactions.

✚ warning: in applying salicylic acid topically, areas of healthy skin and the anogenital region should be avoided. Application to large areas is also inadvisable (absorption through the skin may lead to gastrointestinal disturbance and ringing in the ears). *Related articles:* PHYTEX; PHYTOCIL.

Sandoglobulin (*Sandoz*) is a proprietary preparation of human normal immunoglobulin (HNIG) available only on prescription, used to make up globulin deficiencies in newborn infants. Treatment is by intravenous infusion and may take place over several consecutive days.

✚ warning: see HNIG.

Savloclens (*ICI*) is a proprietary non-prescription ANTISEPTIC used to prevent infection of wounds and burns. Produced in the form of sachets of sterile solution, Savloclens is a compound preparation of the disinfectants chlorhexidine gluconate and cetrimide. It is generally available only in hospitals.

▲/✚ side-effects/warning: *see* CETRIMIDE; CHLORHEXIDINE GLUCONATE.

Savlodil (*ICI*) is a proprietary non-prescription ANTISEPTIC used to prevent infection of wounds and burns. Produced in the form of sachets of sterile solution, Savlodil is a compound preparation of the disinfectants chlorhexidine gluconate and cetrimide. (It is a weaker preparation than the similar Savloclens.)

▲/✚ side-effects/warning: *see* CETRIMIDE; CHLORHEXIDINE GLUCONATE.

Savlon Hospital Concentrate (*ICI*) is a proprietary non-prescription ANTISEPTIC used to prevent infection of wounds and burns, and to prepare skin prior to surgery. Produced in the form of sachets of sterile solution, Savlon Hospital Concentrate is a compound preparation of the disinfectants chlorhexidine gluconate and cetrimide, and may be used in diluted form.

▲/✚ side-effects/warning: *see* CETRIMIDE; CHLORHEXIDINE GLUCONATE.

*scabicidal drugs are used to treat infestations by itch-mites (*Sarcoptes scabiei*). The female mite tunnels into the top surface of the skin in order to lay eggs, causing severe irritation as she does so. Newly-hatched mites, also causing irritation with their secretions, then pass easily from person to person on direct contact. Treatment is (almost always) with local applications of hexachlorophane or benzyl benzoate in the form of a cream: these kill the mites. Every member of an infected household should be treated, and clothing and bedding should also be disinfested.

Securopen (*Bayer*) is a proprietary ANTIBIOTIC of the penicillin type, available only on prescription, used primarily to treat infections of the urinary tract, upper respiratory tract, and septicaemia. Produced in the form of powder in vials for reconstitution as a medium for infusion, Securopen is a preparation of azlocillin.

▲/✚ side-effects/warning: *see* AZLOCILLIN.

Selexid (*Leo*) is a proprietary ANTIBIOTIC of the penicillin type, available only on prescription, used to treat many forms of infection caused by gram-negative bacteria, but particularly salmonellosis and infections of the urinary tract. Produced in the form of tablets and as a suspension (in sachets), Selexid is a preparation of the drug pivmecillinam hydrochloride. It is more rapidly absorbed than mecillinam.

▲/✚ side-effects/warning: *see* PIVMECILLINAM HYDROCHLORIDE.

S

Selexidin (*Leo*) is a proprietary ANTIBIOTIC of the penicillin type, available only on prescription, used to treat many forms of infection caused by gram-negative bacteria, but particularly those of the intestines and the urinary tract. Produced in the form of a powder for reconstitution as a medium for injections, Selexidin is a preparation of the drug mecillinam.

▲/✚ side-effects/warning: *see* MECILLINAM.

Septrin (*Wellcome*) is a proprietary ANTIBIOTIC combination available only on prescription, used to treat bacterial infections, especially of the urinary tract, infections such as sinusitis and bronchitis, and infections of bones and joints. Produced in the form of tablets (in three strengths), as soluble (dispersible) tablets, as a suspension (in two strengths) for dilution (the potency of either suspension once diluted is retained for 14 days), and in ampoules for injection or (following dilution) infusion, Septrin is a preparation of the compound drug co-trimoxazole, made up of the SULPHONAMIDE sulphamethoxazole, with trimethoprim.

▲/✚ side-effects/warning: *see* CO-TRIMOXAZOLE.

silver nitrate is a salt that has astringent and ANTISEPTIC properties useful in topical application to wounds and burns, and is also used as a styptic (to stop bleeding or suppuration) or as a caustic (to cauterize warts). Administration is thus topical, mostly in creams and ointments, or in solution, but also in the form of sticks. In other countries silver nitrate is sometimes used in mild solution in eye-drops.

✚ warning: silver nitrate is toxic if ingested; prolonged application discolours the skin (and fabrics). Solutions should be protected from light.

silver sulphadiazine is a compound ANTIBIOTIC preparation of silver with the SULPHONAMIDE sulphadiazine. In the form of a cream for topical application, it has broad-spectrum ANTIBACTERIAL capability as well as the astringent and ANTISEPTIC qualities of the silver, and is used primarily to inhibit infection of burns and bedsores.

▲ side-effects: side-effects are rare, but there may be sensitivity reactions including rashes.

✚ warning: silver sulphadiazine should not be administered to patients who are allergic to sulphonamides; it should be administered with caution to those with impaired function of the liver or kidneys. *Related article:* FLAMAZINE.

smallpox vaccine is now retained only in specialist centres for researchers working with dangerous viruses (and in a possible emergency on doctors who may be called to treat suspected cases of smallpox) — for smallpox has officially been eradicated. Technically, however, smallpox vaccine is still available on prescription, and consists of a suspension of live (but attenuated) viruses, freeze-dried and supplied with a diluent for reconstitution. Administration is through a short linear scratch, or by "multiple pressure inoculation".

✚ warning: smallpox vaccine should not be administered to patients who are pregnant or aged under 12 months, or with any infection or immune system deficiency.

Sno Phenicol (*Smith & Nephew*) is a proprietary ANTIBIOTIC used to treat bacterial infections. It is a preparation of the potentially toxic drug chloramphenicol.

▲/✚ side-effects/warning: *see* CHLORAMPHENICOL.

sodium fusidate is a narrow-spectrum ANTIBIOTIC used most commonly in combination with other antibiotics to treat staphylococcal infections — especially skin infections, abscesses and infections of bone — that prove to be resistant to penicillin. The drug works by inhibiting protein synthesis at the ribosome level in sensitive organisms (gram-positive bacteria). Administration is oral in the form of tablets and as a suspension, or by infusion.

▲ side-effects: there may be nausea with vomiting; a rash may occur. Some patients experience temporary kidney dysfunction.

✚ warning: regular monitoring of liver function is essential during treatment.
Related article: FUCIDIN.

sodium hypochlorite solutions are used as DISINFECTANTS for cleansing abrasions, burns and ulcers. They differ only in concentration. Non-proprietary solutions are available in 8% and 1% (chlorine) concentrations. Both must be diluted before use, for normal skin can tolerate no more than 0.5% available chlorine in topical application.

sodium perborate is an ANTISEPTIC (and deodorant) powder that is soluble in water. As a mouth-wash the solution has a cleansing effect because it tends to froth on contact with plaque and other oral debris.

✚ warning: sodium perborate should not be used continuously for more than about 4 weeks or borate poisoning may occur.
Related article: BOCASAN.

sodium stibogluconate is an ANTHELMINTIC, used to treat forms of the tropical disease leishmaniasis or kala-azar (caused by parasitic protozoa transmitted in sandfly bites) that leave extensive or unsightly lesions on the skin surface, or that have a similar effect internally. Administration is by slow intravenous injection (which must immediately be halted if there is an attack of coughing or the onset of chest pain), or intramuscular injection (which can be painful).

▲ side-effects: there may be vomiting, coughing and chest pain; continued treatment may lead to severe weight loss (anorexia).

✚ warning: sodium stibogluconate should not be administered to patients with hepatitis, pneumonia, kidney disease or inflammation of the heart.
Related article: PENTOSTAM.

S

Soframycin (*Roussel*) is a proprietary ANTIBIOTIC, available only on prescription, used to treat many forms of infection. Major uses include disinfection of the intestines (especially prior to intestinal surgery), topical application on the skin, injection into the membranes that surround the spinal cord, as eye-drops and eye ointment, and as a cream for use in the outer ear. Produced in the form of tablets, as a powder for reconstitution as a medium for injection or for topical application, as drops, as an ointment and as a water-miscible cream, Soframycin in all forms is a preparation of the broad-spectrum aminoglycoside framycetin sulphate.

▲/✚ side-effects/warning: *see* FRAMYCETIN.

spectinomycin is an ANTIBIOTIC used almost solely to treat gonorrhoea caused by organisms resistant to penicillin, or in patients who are allergic to penicillin. Spectinomycin is related to the aminoglycoside antibiotics both in structure and by the fact that it inhibits protein synthesis in sensitive bacteria by an action on the ribosome. Administration is by injection.

▲ side-effects: there may be nausea with vomiting, high temperature and dizziness; some patients experience urticaria or itching skin.

✚ warning: it is essential that both sexual partners undergo treatment even if only one shows symptoms. (Dosage for women is twice that for men.)

Related article: TROBICIN.

Sporanox (*Janssen*) is a proprietary ANTIFUNGAL preparation, available only on prescription, used for the treatment of vulvovaginal candidiasis and ringworm infections of the scalp, body, feet etc. Administration is oral, in the form of tablets. Sporanox's active ingredient is itraconazole.

▲/✚ side-effects/warning: *see* ITRACONAZOLE.

Stabillin-V-K (*Boots*) is a proprietary preparation of the penicillin-type ANTIBIOTIC phenoxymethylpenicillin, used primarily to treat infections of the ear and throat, and some skin conditions; it may also be used to prevent streptococcal infections in a patient at risk of rheumatic fever. Available only on prescription, it is produced in the form of tablets and as an elixir (in three strengths) for dilution (the potency of the elixir once diluted is retained for 7 days).

▲/✚ side-effects/warning: *see* PHENOXYMETHYLPENICILLIN.

Stafoxil (*Brocades*) is a proprietary ANTIBIOTIC, available only on prescription, used to treat bacterial infections of the skin and of the ear, nose and throat, and especially staphylococcal infections that prove to be resistant to penicillin. Produced in the form of capsules (in two strengths), Stafoxil is a preparation of flucloxacillin. It is not recommended for children aged under 2 years.

▲/✚ side-effects/warning: *see* FLUCLOXACILLIN.

Staphcil (*Lederle*) is a proprietary ANTIBIOTIC, available only on prescription, used to treat bacterial infections and especially staphylococcal infections that prove to be resistant to penicillin. Produced in the form of capsules (in two strengths) and in vials for injection, Staphcil is a preparation of flucloxacillin.

▲/✚ side-effects/warning: *see* FLUCLOXACILLIN.

Steribath (*Stuart*) is a proprietary, non-prescription, concentrated solution for use in the bath as a DISINFECTANT and cleansing agent. Its active constituent is a form of iodine.

Ster-Zac (*Hough*) is the name of three proprietary DISINFECTANT cleansing products. Ster-Zac Powder is a non-prescription dusting powder used to prevent infection in minor wounds and bedsores; it contains the antiseptic hexachlorophane, the mild astringent zinc oxide, and starch. Ster-Zac Bath Concentrate is a mild solution of the antiseptic triclosan, available without prescription, used to treat staphylococcal skin infections. And Ster-Zac DC Skin Cleanser, available only on prescription, is intended for use instead of soap either for surgeons to

S

scrub up with before undertaking surgical operations, or for patients who suffer from acne and skin infections; it contains the antiseptic hexachlorophane in the form of a cream.

▲/✚ side-effects/warning: *see* HEXACHLOROPHANE.

streptomycin is an aminoglycoside ANTIBIOTIC now used almost solely for the treatment of tuberculosis, for which it is administered in combination with other antibiotics. Like other aminoglycosides, streptomycin inhibits protein synthesis in sensitive organisms. Treatment of tuberculosis takes between 6 and 18 months. Administration of streptomycin is by injection. In the rare treatment of urinary and intestinal infections (with or without penicillin) it is administered orally.

✚ warning: streptomycin should not be administered to patients who are pregnant, and should be administered with extreme caution to patients with impaired kidney function. Regular checks on the level of streptomycin in the blood are essential to judge dosage and to guard against toxic levels.

▲ side-effects: there may be hearing difficulties at which the withdrawal of the drug should be considered as irreversible deafness may result from high dosage and/or prolonged treatment; dysfunction of the kidneys may occur in elderly patients. Prolonged treatment may cause an excess of magnesium in the body.

sulconazole nitrate is an ANTIFUNGAL drug, one of the imidazoles, used to treat skin infections. Administration is by topical application in the form of a water-miscible cream.

▲ side-effects: some patients experience sensitivity reactions, especially skin irritation.

✚ warning: keep well away from the eyes.
Related article: EXELDERM.

Suleo-C (*International Labs*) is a proprietary non-prescription drug used to treat infestations of the scalp and pubic hair by lice. Produced in the form of a lotion and a shampoo, Suleo-C is a preparation of the pediculicide carbaryl.

✚warning: see CARBARYL.

Suleo-M (*International Labs*) is a proprietary non-prescription drug used to treat infestations of the scalp and pubic hair by lice (pediculosis), or of the skin by the itch-mite (scabies). Produced in the form of a lotion, Suleo-M is a preparation of the insecticide malathion in an alcohol solution.

✚warning: see MALATHION.

sulfadoxine is an ANTIBIOTIC, a long-acting SULPHONAMIDE, used solely in combination with PYRIMETHAMINE to prevent or treat malaria.

▲side-effects: there may be nausea with vomiting, skin disorders and changes in the composition of the blood.

✚warning: sulfadoxine should not be administered to patients with liver or kidney failure, or blood disorders, who are pregnant, or who are aged under 6 weeks; it should be administered with caution to those who are elderly, or who are lactating. Adequate fluid intake must be maintained; regular blood counts are essential during prolonged treatment.

Related article: KELFIZINE W.

sulfametopyrazine is an ANTIBACTERIAL, a long-acting SULPHONAMIDE, used primarily in the treatment of chronic bronchitis and infections of the urinary tract. Administration is oral in the form of tablets.

▲side-effects: there may be nausea with vomiting, skin disorders and changes in the composition of the blood.

✚warning: sulfametopyrazine should not be administered to patients with liver or kidney failure, or blood disorders, who are pregnant, or who are aged under 6 weeks; it should be administered with caution to those who are elderly, or who are lactating.

S

Adequate fluid intake must be maintained; regular blood counts are essential during prolonged treatment. *Related article:* KELFIZINE W.

sulphacetamide is an ANTIBIOTIC, one of the SULPHONAMIDES, used (in solution) primarily in the form of eye-drops and eye ointment to treat local bacterial infections. However, it is no longer recommended for this purpose as there are other more effective drugs. It is also used in combination with other sulphonamides to treat infections of the vagina and cervix. Ophthalmic administration is most commonly in the form of drops during the daytime, and as ointment for overnight treatment; treatment for vaginal infections is in the form of vaginal tablets (pessaries) or as a cream.

S

sulphadiazine is an ANTIBIOTIC, one of the SULPHONAMIDES, used to treat serious bacterial infections − particularly meningococcal meningitis. Administration is oral in the form of tablets, or by infusion.

▲ side-effects: there may be nausea and vomiting, with skin disorders; changes in the composition of the blood may occur.

✚ warning: sulphadiazine should not be administered to patients with liver or kidney failure, or disorders of the blood, who are pregnant, or who are aged under 6 weeks; it should be administered with caution to those with impaired kidney function or sensitivity to light, who are elderly, or who are lactating. Adequate fluid intake is essential to avoid the risk of the drug crystallizing out in the urine. Regular blood counts should be done during prolonged courses of treatment.

sulphadimethoxine is a long-acting ANTIBIOTIC, one of the SULPHONAMIDES, used to treat the eye disorder trachoma, which is common in underdeveloped countries. Administration is oral in the form of tablets. It is not marketed in the United Kingdom.

▲ side-effects: there may be nausea and vomiting, with skin disorders; changes in the composition of the blood may occur.

✚ warning: sulphadimethoxine should not be administered to patients with liver or kidney failure, or disorders of the blood, who are pregnant, or who are aged under 6 weeks; it should be administered with caution to those with impaired kidney function or sensitivity to light, who are elderly, or who are lactating. Adequate fluid intake is essential, as are regular blood counts during prolonged courses of treatment.

Related article: MADRIBON.

sulphadimidine is an ANTIBIOTIC, one of the SULPHONAMIDES, used to treat serious bacterial infections — particularly infections of the urinary tract — and to prevent meningococcal meningitis in patients at high risk from infection. Among the least toxic of the sulphonamides, sulphadimidine is especially useful in the treatment of children. Administration is oral in the form of tablets, or by injection.

✚ warning: sulphadimidine should not be administered to patients who suffer from liver or kidney failure, or disorders of the blood, who are pregnant, or who are aged under 6 weeks; it should be administered with caution to those with impaired kidney function or sensitivity to light, who are elderly, or who are lactating. Adequate fluid intake is essential, as are regular blood counts during prolonged courses of treatment.

▲ side-effects: there may be nausea and vomiting, with skin disorders; changes in the composition of the blood may occur.

Related article: SULPHAMEZATHINE.

sulphaguanidine is an ANTIBIOTIC, one of the SULPHONAMIDES, formerly in widespread use to treat intestinal infections or to prepare patients for intestinal surgery (because absorption into the body is poor and does not occur early in the digestive processes). Administration is oral in the form of (non-proprietary) tablets. However, other more effective drugs are now recommended for these situations.

▲ side-effects: there may be nausea and vomiting, with frequent skin rashes; changes in the composition of the blood may occur.

✚ warning: sulphaguanidine should not be administered to patients with liver or kidney failure, or disorders of the blood, who are pregnant, or who are aged under 6 weeks; it should be administered with caution to those with impaired kidney function or sensitivity to light, who are elderly, or who are lactating. Adequate fluid intake is essential, as are regular blood counts during prolonged courses of treatment.

sulphamethoxazole is an ANTIBIOTIC, one of the SULPHONAMIDES, that in combination with another antibiotic agent TRIMETHOPRIM — forming a compound drug called co-trimoxazole — is in widespread use to treat many serious infections, especially infections of the bones and joints, or the urinary tract and of the upper respiratory tract, and such infections as gonorrhoea and typhoid fever. Rarely, sulphamethoxazole is used by itself in the treatment of urinary infections; administration is oral in the form of tablets, and patients should be advised to increase fluid intake during treatment.
Related article: CO-TRIMOXAZOLE.

Sulphamezathine (*ICI*) is a proprietary ANTIBIOTIC, available only on prescription, used to treat serious bacterial infections — particularly bacillary dysentery and infections of the urinary tract — and to prevent meningococcal meningitis in patients at high risk from infection. Produced in ampoules for injection, Sulphamezathine is a preparation of the SULPHONAMIDE sulphadimidine.

▲/✚ side-effects/warning: *see* SULPHADIMIDINE.

sulphaurea is an ANTIBACTERIAL, one of the SULPHONAMIDES, used to treat infections of the urinary tract, although it is no longer recommended. Administration is oral in the form of tablets (generally also containing the analgesic phenazopyridine).

▲ side-effects: there may be nausea and vomiting, with skin disorders; changes in the composition of the blood may occur.

✚ warning: sulphaurea should not be administered to patients with liver or kidney failure, or disorders of the blood, who are pregnant, or who are aged under 6 weeks; it should be administered with caution to those with impaired kidney function or sensitivity to light, who are elderly, or who are lactating. Adequate fluid intake is essential, as are regular blood counts during prolonged courses of treatment.

Related article: UROMIDE.

sulphonamides are derivatives of a red dye called sulphanilamide that have the property of preventing the growth of bacteria. They were the first group of drugs with general utility as antibiotic agents. Their antibacterial action stems from their chemical similarity to a compound required by bacteria to generate the essential growth factor, folic acid. This similarity inhibits the production of folic acid by bacteria (and therefore growth) while the human host is able to utilize folic acid in the diet. Most are administered orally and are rapidly absorbed in the stomach and small intestine, are short-acting, and thus may have to be taken several times a day. Their quick progress through the body and excretion in the urine makes them particularly suited to the treatment of urinary infections. One or two sulphonamides are long-acting (and may be used to treat diseases such as malaria or leprosy), and another one or two are poorly absorbed (for which reason they were until recently used to treat intestinal infections). Best known and most used sulphonamides include sulphadiazine, sulphadimidine and sulfametopyrazine. Sulphonamides tend to cause side-effects – particularly nausea, vomiting, diarrhoea and headache − some of which (especially sensitivity reactions) may become serious; bone-marrow damage may result from prolonged treatment. Such serious hypersensitivity reactions are more of a risk with the longer-acting sulphonamides, which can accumulate in the body. As a general rule, patients being treated with sulphonamides should try to avoid exposure to sunlight. In general the sulphonamides are being replaced by newer antibiotics with greater activity, fewer problems with bacterial resistance and less risk of side-effects.

see SULFADOXINE; SULFAMETOPYRAZINE; SULPHACETAMIDE; SULPHADIAZINE; SULPHADIMETHOXINE; SULPHADIMIDINE; SULPHAGUANIDINE; SULPHAMETHOXAZOLE; SULPHAUREA.

sulphones are closely related to the SULPHONAMIDES, have much the same therapeutic action, and are thus used for much the same purposes. They are particularly successful in preventing the growth of the bacteria responsible for leprosy, malaria and tuberculosis. Best known and (possibly) most used is dapsone.

see DAPSONE.

Sultrin (*Ortho-Cilag*) is a proprietary ANTIBOTIC, available only on prescription, used to treat bacterial infections of the vagina or the cervix, or to prevent infection following gynaecological surgery. Produced in the form of vaginal tablets (pessaries) and as a cream (with its own applicator), Sultrin is a compound of three SULPHONAMIDE antibacterial agents: sulphacetamide, sulphabenzamide and sulphathiazole.

suramin is a powerful drug that has been used in the treatment of infestations by filaria (threadlike nematode worms that parasitize the connective and lymphatic tissues of the body following transmission through the bite of a bloodsucking insect). On account of its toxicity it has been largely replaced by more effective and less toxic agents. It is also used to treat the early stages of trypanosomiasis (a tropical protozoal infection such as sleeping sickness, transmitted through bites of the tsetse fly). Administration is initially by infusion, and then by injection.

✚ warning: suramin is toxic to the kidneys; a course of treatment lasts a maximum of 5 weeks, and regular urine analysis is essential.

Sustamycin (*MCP Pharmaceuticals*) is a proprietary broad-spectrum ANTIBIOTIC, available only on prescription, used to treat many forms of infection. Produced in the form of sustained-release capsules, Sustamycin is a preparation of tetracycline hydrochloride. It is not recommended for children.

▲/✚ side-effects/warning: *see* TETRACYCLINE.

Syraprim (*Wellcome*) is a proprietary ANTIBIOTIC drug, available only on prescription, used to treat serious bacterial infections, particularly those of the upper respiratory tract and of the urinary tract. Produced in the form of tablets (in two strengths) and in ampoules for injection, Syraprim is a preparation of the antibacterial agent trimethoprim.

▲/✚ side-effects/warning: *see* TRIMETHOPRIM.

S

talampicillin is a broad-spectrum penicillin-type ANTIBIOTIC, a more readily absorbed derivative of ampicillin, used to treat various bacterial infections (such as chronic bronchitis, gonorrhoea, infection of the middle ear, and infections of the urinary tract). Administration is oral in the form of tablets and as a dilute syrup.

▲ side-effects: there may be sensitivity reactions. Some patients experience diarrhoea.

✚ warning: talampicillin should not be administered to patients known to be sensitive to penicillins; it should be administered with caution to those with any allergy at all, or to those with impaired kidney function.
Related article: TALPEN.

Talpen (*Beecham*) is a proprietary ANTIBIOTIC of the penicillin type, available only on prescription, used to treat severe bacterial infections (such as chronic bronchitis, gonorrhoea, infection of the middle ear, and infections of the urinary tract). Produced in the form of tablets, and as a syrup for dilution (the potency of the syrup once diluted is retained for 7 days), Talpen is a preparation of the ampicillin-derivative talampicillin.

▲/✚ side-effects/warning: *see* TALAMPICILLIN.

Terramycin (*Pfizer*) is a proprietary ANTIBIOTIC, available only on prescription, used to treat bacterial and other infections. Produced in the form of capsules and tablets, it is a preparation of the TETRACYCLINE oxytetracycline hydrochloride.

▲/✚ side-effects/warning: *see* OXYTETRACYCLINE.

tetanus vaccine is a toxoid VACCINE that stimulates the formation in the body of the appropriate antitoxin — that is, an antibody produced in response to the presence of the toxin of the tetanus bacterium, rather than to the presence of the bacterium itself. Its effectiveness is improved by being adsorbed on to a mineral carrier (such as aluminium hydroxide or calcium phosphate). Its most common form of administration is as one constituent of the triple vaccine against diphtheria, whooping cough (pertussis) and tetanus (the DIPHTHERIA-PERTUSSIS-TETANUS, or DPT, vaccine), administered during early life, although it is administered by itself at any age for those at special risk, or administered as a double vaccine with the DIPHTHERIA VACCINE for those who wish not to be given the whooping cough vaccine. Administration is by injection. Tetanus vaccinations should not be renewed within 5 years.

Tetavax (*Merieux*) is a proprietary preparation of adsorbed TETANUS VACCINE, produced in syringes and vials for injection.

tet/vac/ads is an abbreviation for the kind of tetanus vaccine that is adsorbed on to a mineral carrier for injection. *see* TETANUS VACCINE.

tet/vac/ft is an abbreviation for tetanus vaccine formol toxoid, the plain vaccine (that is not adsorbed on to a carrier).
see TETANUS VACCINE.

Tetrabid-Organon (*Organon*) is a proprietary broad-spectrum ANTIBIOTIC, available only on prescription, used to treat many forms of infection but particularly those of the urinary tract, of the genital organs, pustular acne or chronic bronchitis. Produced in the form of sustained-release capsules, it is a preparation of the TETRACYCLINE tetracycline hydrochloride. It is not suitable for children aged under 12 years.
▲/✚ side-effects/warning: *see* TETRACYCLINE.

Tetrachel (*Berk*) is a proprietary broad-spectrum ANTIBIOTIC, available only on prescription, used to treat many forms of infection but particularly those of the urinary tract, of the genital organs, pustular acne or chronic bronchitis. Produced in the form of capsules and tablets, it is a preparation of the TETRACYCLINE tetracycline hydrochloride. It is not suitable for children aged under 12 years.
▲/✚ side-effects/warning: *see* TETRACYCLINE.

tetracycline is a broad-spectrum ANTIBIOTIC that gave its name to a group of similar antibiotics. It is used to treat many forms of infection caused by several types of micro-organism; conditions it is used to treat include infections of the urinary tract, of the respiratory tract, and of the genital organs, and acne. Administration is oral in the form of capsules, tablets and liquids, or by injection.

▲ side-effects: there may be nausea and vomiting, with diarrhoea. Occasionally there is sensitivity to light or other sensitivity reaction. These side-effects may still occur even if the causative organism of the disorder being treated proves to be resistant to the drug.

✚ warning: tetracycline should not be administered to patients who are aged under 12 years, who are pregnant, or who have impaired kidney function; it should be administered with caution to those who are lactating.

Related articles: ACHROMYCIN; ACHROMYCIN V; AUREOCORT; CHYMOCYCLAR; DETECLO; ECONOMYCIN; MYSTECLIN; SUSTAMYCIN; TETRABID-ORGANON; TETRACHEL; TETREX; TOPICYCLINE.

tetracyclines are a group of very broad-spectrum ANTIBIOTICS. Apart from being effective against bacteria, they inhibit the growth of chlamydia (cause genito-urinary tract infections, eye infections and psittacosis), rickettsia (cause Q fever and typhus) and mycoplasma (cause mycoplasmal pneumonia). They act by inhibiting protein biosynthesis in sensitive micro-organisms and penetrate human macrophages, therefore they are useful in combating micro-organisms such as mycoplasma that can survive and multiply within macrophages. They have been used to treat a very wide range of infections, but with developing bacterial resistance their uses have become more specific. Treatment of atypical pneumonia due to chlamydia, rickettsia or mycoplasma is a notable indication for tetracyclines, while treatment of chlamydial urethritis and pelvic inflammatory disease is another. They are also used to treat brucellosis and Lyme disease. More mundanely they are effective in treating exacerbations of chronic bronchitis. Most tetracyclines are more difficult to absorb in a stomach that contains milk, antacids, calcium salts or magnesium salts; they tend to make kidney disease worse; and they may be deposited in growing bone and teeth (causing staining and potential deformity), so they should not be administered to children aged under 12 years. Best known and most used tetracyclines include tetracycline (which they were all named after), doxycycline and oxytetracycline. Administration is oral in the form of capsules, tablets or liquids.

see CHLORTETRACYCLINE HYDROCHLORIDE; CLOMOCYCLINE SODIUM; DEMECLOCYCLINE HYDROCHLORIDE; DOXYCYCLINE; LYMECYCLINE; MINOCYCLINE; OXYTETRACYCLINE; TETRACYCLINE.

Tetralysal (*Farmitalia Carlo Erba*) is a proprietary broad-spectrum ANTIBIOTIC, available only on prescription, used to treat many forms of infection but particularly those of the skin and soft tissues, the ear, nose or throat, or conditions such as pustular acne. Produced in the form of capsules (in two strengths, the stronger under the name Tetralysal 300), it represents a preparation of the soluble TETRACYCLINE complex lymecycline. It is not recommended for children aged under 12 years.

▲/✚ side-effects/warning: *see* LYMECYCLINE.

Tetrex (*Bristol-Myers*) is a proprietary broad-spectrum ANTIBIOTIC, available only on prescription, used to treat many forms of infection but particularly those of the urinary tract or genital organs, pustular acne or chronic bronchitis. Produced in the form of capsules and tablets, it is a preparation of tetracycline hydrochloride. It is not recommended for children aged under 12 years.

▲/✚ side-effects/warning: *see* TETRACYCLINE.

Ticar (*Beecham*) is a proprietary ANTIBIOTIC, available only on prescription, used to treat serious infections such as septicaemia and peritonitis, in addition to infections of the respiratory tract or urinary tract. It may also be used to prevent infection in wounds. Produced in the form of a powder for reconstitution as a medium for injection, and in infusion bottles, Ticar is a preparation of the penicillin ticarcillin sodium.

▲/✚ side-effects/warning: *see* TICARCILLIN.

ticarcillin is an ANTIBIOTIC, one of the penicillins with improved activity against a number of important gram-negative bacteria including *Pseudomonas aeruginosa*. It is used to treat serious infections such as septicaemia and peritonitis, in addition to infections of the respiratory tract or of the urinary tract. It may also be used to prevent infection in wounds. Administration is by injection or infusion.

▲ side-effects: there may be sensitivity reactions ranging from a minor rash to urticaria and joint pains, and (occasionally) to high temperature or anaphylactic shock.

✚ warning: ticarcillin should not be administered to patients known to be allergic to penicillins; it should be administered with caution to those with impaired kidney function.

Related articles: TICAR; TIMENTIN.

Tiempe (*DDSA Pharmaceuticals*) is a proprietary ANTIBIOTIC, available only on prescription, used primarily to treat infections of the urinary or respiratory tracts, and especially bronchitis. Produced in the form of tablets (in two strengths), it is a preparation of the antibacterial agent trimethoprim.

▲/✚ side-effects/warning: *see* TRIMETHOPRIM.

Timentin (*Beecham*) is a proprietary ANTIBIOTIC, available only on prescription, used to treat severe infections in patients whose immune systems are undermined by disease or drugs, and where the responsible micro-organism is resistant to ticarcillin alone because it produces a penicillinase enzyme that destroys ticarcillin. (Patients with such conditions are generally in hospital.) Produced in the form of a powder for reconstitution as a medium for injection, Timentin is a compound

preparation of the pencillinase enzyme inhibitor
clavulanic acid with the penicillin ticarcillin.
▲/✚ side-effects/warning: *see* TICARCILLIN.

Timoped (*Reckitt & Colman*) is a proprietary non-prescription cream for topical application to fungal skin
infections (such as athlete's foot). Intended to be
massaged into the affected area and allowed to dry to a
white powder, the cream is a preparation of the
ANTIFUNGAL drug TOLNAFTATE with the ANTISEPTIC TRICLOSAN.

Tinaderm-M (*Kirby-Warrick*) is a proprietary non-prescription cream for topical application to fungal
infections of the skin and nails. Intended to be applied
two or three times a day, the cream is a preparation of
the ANTIFUNGAL drugs TOLNAFTATE and nystatin.
▲/✚ side-effects/warning: *see* NYSTATIN.

Tineafax (*Wellcome*) is a proprietary non-prescription
ointment for topical application to fungal skin infections
(such as athlete's foot). It is a preparation of two ANTIFUNGAL
zinc salts. A powdered form containing zinc salt is also
available for use as a dusting-powder in a puffer pack, and
is intended to prevent fungal skin infection.

tinidazole is an ANTIBIOTIC active against anaerobic
bacteria; it also has ANTIPROTOZOAL activity. It resembles
metronidazole and, like it, is used to treat anaerobic
infections throughout the body and protozoal infections
such as giardiasis, trichomoniasis and amoebiasis. It may
also be used to treat acute ulcerative gingivitis.
Administration is oral in the form of tablets, or by
intravenous infusion.
▲ side-effects: there may be nausea and vomiting, with
gastrointestinal disturbance; drowsiness and headache
may occur. Less commonly, there may be a rash,
discoloration of the urine, tingling or numbness of the
extremities and a reduction in white cells in the blood.
High doses in susceptible patients may bring on
epilepsy-like seizures.

T

✚warning: tinidazole should be administered with caution to patients with impaired liver function, or who are pregnant or lactating. On no account should alcohol be consumed during treatment (for even a small amount can cause severe reaction).
Related article: FASIGYN.

tioconazole is a synthetic ANTIFUNGAL drug of the imidazole family, used principally in the topical treatment of infection by the tinea species known as ringworm (such as athlete's foot). Administration is in the form of a solution. To be effective treatment must be continued for more than six months. Rarely sensitivity reactions occur.

Tisept (*Schering*) is a DISINFECTANT used mainly for surgical procedures in obstetrics or in dressing wounds and burns. Produced in sachets and in bottles, it is a compound solution of the two ANTISEPTICS CHLORHEXIDINE gluconate and CETRIMIDE.

Tobralex (*Alcon*) is a proprietary preparation of the aminoglycoside ANTIBIOTIC tobramycin, available only on prescription, used in the form of eye-drops to treat bacterial infections of the eye.
▲/✚ side-effects/warning: *see* TOBRAMYCIN.

tobramycin is an ANTIBIOTIC, one of the aminoglycosides, effective against some gram-positive and gram-negative bacteria. It is used primarily for the treatment of serious gram-negative infections caused by *Pseudomonas aeruginosa* as it is significantly more active against this organism than gentamicin (the most commonly used of this class of antibiotic). Like other aminoglycosides it is not absorbed from the intestine (except in the case of local infection or liver failure) and so is administered by injection when treating systemic disease. It is also produced in the form of eye-drops to treat bacterial infections of the eye.
▲ side-effects: treatment must be discontinued if there are any signs of deafness. There may be dysfunction of the kidneys.

✚ warning: tobramycin should not be administered to patients who are pregnant, or who are already taking drugs that affect the neural system. It should be administered with caution to those with parkinsonism or impaired kidney function. Prolonged or high dosage can cause deafness; regular blood level checks are essential in such cases.
Related articles: NEBCIN; TOBRALEX.

tolnaftate is a mild, synthetic, ANTIFUNGAL drug used principally in the topical treatment of infections by the Tinea species known as ringworm (such as athlete's foot). Administration is in the form of a cream, a powder or a solution. Rarely, sensitivity reactions occur.
Related article: TIMOPED; TINADERM-N.

Topicycline (*Norwich Eaton*) is a proprietary ANTIBIOTIC, available only on prescription, used to treat acne. Produced in the form of a solution for topical application, it is a preparation of the tetracycline hydrochloride, and is not recommended for children.
▲/✚ side-effects/warning: *see* TETRACYCLINE.

Travasept (*Travenol*) is a proprietary non-prescription DISINFECTANT for use in cleaning wounds and burns. Produced in sachets of solution (not for further dilution), Travasept is a compound preparation of the antiseptics cetrimide and chlorhexidine acetate (in two strengths, under the trade names Travasept 30 and Travasept 100).

Travogyn (*Schering*) is a proprietary ANTIFUNGAL drug, available only on prescription, used in the treatment of fungal or fungal-and-bacterial infections of the vagina or the ano-genital area. Produced in the form of a cream for topical application, and as vaginal tablets (pessaries), it is a preparation of isoconazole nitrate.
▲ side-effects: see ISOCONAZOLE.

Tribiotic (*Riker*) is a proprietary ANTIBIOTIC, available only on prescription, used as a spray in topical

T

application to infections of the skin. Produced in aerosol units, it is a compound preparation of three antibiotics: neomycin sulphate, polymyxin B sulphate and bacitracin zinc.

triclosan is a mildly ANTIBIOTIC DISINFECTANT for topical application to the skin. It is sometimes used to treat staphylococcal infection, but it is primarily used to prevent the spread of infection within hospitals or households. It should be kept away from the eyes.
Related articles: MANUSEPT; STER-ZAC; TIMOPED.

trimethoprim is an ANTIBIOTIC agent similar in action to the sulphonamides, used to treat and to prevent the spread of many forms of bacterial infection but particularly those of the urinary and respiratory tracts. It has been used particularly in combination with a SULPHONAMIDE drug, for the combined effect has been thought to be greater than twice the individual effect of either partner. This is the basis of the medicinal compound co-trimoxazole (which forms the active constituent of many proprietary preparations). More recently there has been a move away from the compound preparation to the use of trimethoprim alone. It is effective in many situations and lacks the side-effects of the sulphonamide present in co-trimoxazole. Administration of trimethoprim is oral in the form of tablets or a dilute suspension, or by injection.

▲ side-effects: there may be nausea, vomiting and gastrointestinal disturbances; rashes may break out, with itching (pruritus).

✚ warning: trimethoprim should not be administered to newborn babies, or to patients who are pregnant, or who have severely impaired kidney function. Dosage should be reduced for patients with poor kidney function. Prolonged therapy requires frequent blood counts.
Related articles: IPRAL; MONOTRIM; SYRAPRIM; TIEMPE; TRIMOGAL; TRIMOPAN.
see also CO-TRIMOXAZOLE.

Trimogal (*Lagap*) is a proprietary ANTIBIOTIC, available only on prescription, used to treat and to prevent the spread of many forms of bacterial infection but particularly those of the urinary and respiratory tracts. Produced in the form of tablets (in two strengths), it is a preparation of the drug trimethoprim.

▲/✚ side-effects/warning: *see* TRIMETHOPRIM.

Trimopan (*Berk*) is a proprietary ANTIBIOTIC agent, available only on prescription, used to treat and to prevent the spread of many forms of bacterial infection, but particularly those of the urinary and respiratory tracts. Produced in the form of tablets (in two strengths), and as a sugar-free suspension for dilution (the potency of the suspension once diluted is retained for 14 days), it is a preparation of the drug trimethoprim.

▲/✚ side-effects/warning: *see* TRIMETHOPRIM.

Triplopen (*Glaxo*) is a proprietary ANTIBIOTIC, used in the treatment or prevention of many forms of bacterial infection. Produced in the form of powder for reconstitution as a medium for injection, it is a compound preparation of three penicillin-type antibiotics: benzylpenicillin sodium, procaine penicillin and benethamine penicillin. The particular asset of this preparation is that following intramuscular injection it creates a depot of forms of penicillin with varying solubilties, from which penicillin is released into the blood over a period many days, thus avoiding the need for frequent injections.

▲/✚ side-effects/warning: *see* BENETHAMINE PENICILLIN; BENZYLPENICILLIN; PROCAINE PENICILLIN.

Trivax (*Wellcome*) is a proprietary preparation of the triple vaccine diphtheria-pertussis-tetanus (DPT) vaccine, consisting of a combination of the toxoids (antibodies produced in response to the toxins) of the diphtheria and tetanus bacteria with pertussis vaccine. It is produced in ampoules for injection.

see DIPHTHERIA-PERTUSSIS-TETANUS (DPT) VACCINE.

Trivax-AD (*Wellcome*) is a proprietary preparation of the triple vaccine diphtheria-pertussis-tetanus (DPT) vaccine, consisting of a combination of the toxoids (antibodies produced in response to the toxins) of the diphtheria and tetanus bacteria with pertussis vaccine, all adsorbed on to a mineral carrier (in the form of aluminium hydroxide). It is produced in ampoules for injection.
see DIPHTHERIA-PERTUSSIS-TETANUS (DPT) VACCINE.

Trobicin (*Upjohn*) is a proprietary ANTIBIOTIC, available only on prescription, used specifically in the treatment of the sexually transmitted disease gonorrhoea in patients who are allergic to penicillins, or in cases resistant to penicillins. Produced in the form of a powder for reconstitution as a medium for injection, it is a preparation of spectinomycin.
▲/✚ side-effects/warning: *see* SPECTINOMYCIN.

Trosyl (*Pfizer*) is a proprietary ANTIFUNGAL preparation available only on prescription for topical application to fungal infections of the nails. Produced in the form of a solution with an applicator brush. Trosyl is a preparation of the antifungal drug tioconazole.
▲/✚ side-effects/warning: *see* TIOCONAZOLE.

tub/vac/BCG, dried, is an abbreviation for the freeze-dried version of BCG VACCINE (against tuberculosis).
see BCG VACCINE.

tub/vac/BCG, perc, is an abbreviation for the live version of BCG VACCINE (against tuberculosis) for percutaneous administration by multiple puncture with a suitable instrument.
see BCG VACCINE.

typhoid vaccine is a suspension of dead typhoid bacteria, administered by deep subcutaneous or intramuscular injection. Full protection is, however, not guaranteed, and travellers at risk are advised not to eat uncooked food or to drink untreated water. Dosage is normally repeated after 4 to 6 weeks – unless reactions have been severe. Some reaction is to be expected: swelling, pain and tenderness occur after a couple of hours, followed by high temperature and malaise, possibly with a headache.

typhus vaccine is not normally available in the United Kingdom, although there are small stocks that can be used if necessary. It consists of inactivated Rickettsia organisms grown in the yolk-sacs of hens' eggs. The organisms are carried by body lice, but good hygienic conditions, in any part of the world, even where the disease is endemic, are usually enough for protection.

Unimycin (*Unigreg*) is a proprietary ANTIBIOTIC, available only on prescription, containing oxytetracycline hydrochloride; it is administered in the form of capsules, and is effective against a wide range of infections.
▲/✚ side-effects/warning: *see* OXYTETRACYCLINE.

Unisept (*Schering*) is a proprietary non-prescription DISINFECTANT and wound cleanser that is available in sachets; each sachet contains chlorhexidine gluconate in very dilute solution.
▲/✚ side-effects/warning: *see* CHLORHEXIDINE.

Urantoin (*DDSA Pharmaceuticals*) is a proprietary form of the ANTIBIOTIC drug nitrofurantoin, used specifically to treat infections of the urinary tract. Produced as tablets, Urantoin is available only on prescription.
▲/✚ side-effects/warning: *see* NITROFURANTOIN.

Uriben (*RP Drugs*) is a proprietary ANTIBIOTIC agent, available only on prescription, in the form of a syrupy suspension of nalidixic acid. Used in solution to treat gastrointestinal infections and infections of the urinary tract, once made up its potency is retained for 14 days.
▲/✚ side-effects/warning: *see* NALIDIXIC ACID.

Uromide (*Consolidated*) is a proprietary SULPHONAMIDE ANTIBIOTIC, available only on prescription, in the form of tablets containing sulphaurea and phenazopyridine hydrochloride. Uromide is used to treat infections of the urinary tract, and apart from its antibacterial properties also has soothing and alkalinizing effects.
▲/✚ side-effects/warning: *see* SULPHAUREA.

Uro-Tainer (*CliniMed*) is the proprietary name for a selection of solutions designed to wash and maintain a latex or silicone catheter replacing or assisting part of the urinary tract. Solutions − available without prescription in the form of sachets − include CHLORHEXIDINE 0.02%; saline (sodium chloride) 0.9%; mandelic acid 1%; and some proprietary compounds.

Uticillin (*Beecham*) is a proprietary ANTIBIOTIC drug, available only on prescription, in the form of tablets containing carfecillin sodium. The tablets are prescribed to treat infections of the urinary tract.

▲/✚ side-effects/warning: *see* CARFECILLIN SODIUM.

*vaccines confer active immunity against specific diseases: that is, they cause a patient's own body to create a defence (in the form of antibodies against the disease). Most are administered in the form of a suspension of dead viruses (as in flu vaccine) or bacteria (as in typhoid vaccine), or of live but weakened viruses (as in rubella vaccine) or bacteria (as in BCG vaccine against tuberculosis). A third type is a suspension containing extracts of the toxins released by the invading organism that stimulates the formation of antibodies against the toxin, not the organism itself. This is called a toxoid vaccine. Vaccines that incorporate dead micro-organisms generally require a series of administrations (most often three) to build up a sufficient supply of antibodies in the body; booster shots may thereafter be necessary at regular intervals to reinforce immunity. Vaccines that incorporate live micro-organisms may confer immunity with a single dose, because the organisms multiply within the body, although some live vaccines still require 3 administrations (as in oral poliomyelitis vaccine).

▲ side-effects: side-effects range from little or no reactions to severe discomfort, high temperature and pain.

✚ warning: vaccination should not be administered to patients who have a febrile illness or any form of infection. Vaccines containing live material should not be administered routinely to patients who are pregnant, or who are known to have an immunodeficiency disorder.

Vancocin (*Lilly*) is the name of a selection of proprietary forms of the antibacterial ANTIBIOTIC vancomycin hydrochloride. Available only on prescription, there are capsules (produced under the name Matrigel) and powdered forms for use in solution orally and as injections.

▲/✚ side-effects/warning: *see* VANCOMYCIN.

vancomycin is an ANTIBIOTIC with activity primarily against gram-positive micro-organisms. It inhibits the synthesis of components of the bacterial cell wall. As it is rather toxic, particularly to the kidneys and ears, it is only used in special situations. One is the treatment of pseudomembranous colitis, a superinfection of the gastrointestinal tract, which can occur after treatment with broad-spectrum antibiotics such as ampicillin or clindamycin. Another use is in the treatment of multiple-drug-resistant staphylococcal infections, particularly endocarditis. It is not absorbed orally but is taken by mouth to treat colitis and by infusion for systemic infections. Because incautious use may have deleterious effects on the organs of the ear, on the kidney, and on the tissues at the site of injection, blood concentrations and tests on liver and kidney functions are necessary during treatment.

▲ side-effects: infusion may cause high body temperature and a rash; incautious use may lead to ringing in the ears (tinnitus) and to kidney disease.

✚ warning: vancomycin should not be administered to patients with impaired kidney function or who are deaf; or to patients in whom there is a risk of the escape of body fluids from the vessels into the tissues. *Related article:* VANCOCIN.

Vansil is a proprietary form of the ANTHELMINTIC drug OXAMNIQUINE, used specifically as an oral treatment for intestinal schistosomiasis (bilharziasis).

var/vac is an abbreviation for variola vaccine. *see* SMALLPOX VACCINE.

V-Cil-K (*Lilly*) is a proprietary preparation of the penicillin-type ANTIBIOTIC phenoxymethylpenicillin, used mainly to treat infections of the ears and throat, and some skin conditions. Available only on prescription, it is produced in the form of capsules, tablets (in two strengths), a syrup for dilution, and a children's syrup (in two strengths) for dilution (the potency of the diluted syrup is retained for 7 days).

▲/✚ side-effects/warning: *see* PHENOXYMETHYLPENICILLIN.

Velosef (*Squibb*) is a proprietary form of the
CEPHALOSPORIN ANTIBIOTIC cephradine, available only on
prescription, as capsules (in two strengths), a syrup (for
dilution) or a powdered form for use in solution as
injections. The potency of the syrup once diluted is
retained for 7 days.
▲/✚ side-effects/warning: *see* CEPHRADINE.

Vermox (*Janssen*) is a proprietary ANTHELMINTIC drug,
available only on prescription, used to treat infestation
by pinworms (threadworms) and similar intestinal
parasites. Consisting of mebendazole, Vermox is
produced in two forms: as tablets and in suspension.
▲/✚ side-effects/warning: *see* MEBENDAZOLE.

Vibramycin (*Pfizer*) is a proprietary form of the
TETRACYCLINE ANTIBIOTIC doxycycline, available only on
prescription, as capsules (in two strengths), a sugar-free
syrup (for dilution) or − under the separate name
Vibramycin-D − soluble (dispersible) tablets. Vibramycin
is prescribed to treat a wide range of bacterial and
microbial infections.
▲/✚ side-effects/warning: *see* DOXYCYCLINE.

vidarabine is an ANTIVIRAL drug used to treat serious
infections by herpes viruses (such as chickenpox and
shingles) in patients whose immune systems are already
suppressed by other drugs. The drug's usefulness is limited
by its toxicity. Administration is by intravenous infusion.
▲ side-effects: there may be nausea and vomiting,
diarrhoea and/or anorexia; a tremor may become
apparent, with dizziness or a state of confusion; in the
blood, white cells and platelets may decrease.
✚ warning: careful monitoring of blood count and kidney
function is required: dosage should be balanced at an
optimum. Treatment with vidarabine is not suitable
for pregnant or lactating women.
Related article: VIRA-A.

Videne (*Riker*) is a proprietary non-prescription skin

disinfectant and cleanser containing povidone-iodine. Much used in hospitals, several forms are available: a water-based solution, a detergent-based surgical scrub, a tincture in methylated spirit (for washing skin preparatory to surgery), and dusting powder (for direct application to minor wounds).

▲/✚ side-effects/warning: *see* POVIDONE-IODINE.

Vidopen (*Berk*) is a proprietary ANTIBIOTIC preparation of the broad-spectrum penicillin called ampicillin, available only on prescription. It is used mainly to treat infections of the respiratory passages, the middle ear and the urinary tract. It is also effective against gonorrhoea. Vidopen is produced as capsules (in two strengths) and as a syrup (in two strengths, for dilution); the potency of the syrup once diluted is retained for 7 days.

▲/✚ side-effects/warning: *see* AMPICILLIN.

Vira-A (*Parke-Davis*) is a proprietary ANTIVIRAL drug, available only on prescription, used to treat herpes infections. It is produced in two forms: as a concentrated fluid for dilution before intravenous infusion or injection, and as an eye ointment. In both cases the active constituent is vidarabine.

▲/✚ side-effects/warning: *see* VIDARABINE.

Virudox (*Ferring*) is a proprietary ANTIVIRAL drug available only on prescription, used to treat infections of the skin by herpes simplex (cold sores, fever sores) or by herpes zoster (shingles). Its effectiveness is enhanced if treatment begins early. Produced in the form of a lotion or paint, for topical application with a brush, Virudox is a solution of idoxuridine in the organic solvent dimethyl sulphoxide (DMSO).

✚ warning: see IDOXURIDINE.

yellow fever vaccine consists of a protein suspension containing live but weakened yellow fever viruses (cultured in chick embryos). Immunity may last for a good deal longer than the official ten years. The disease remains relatively well established in parts of tropical Africa and northern South America.

▲ side-effects: reactions are rare.

✚ warning: vaccination should not be administered to patients with an impaired immune response; who are sensitive to eggs; who are pregnant; or who are aged under 9 months.

Related articles: ARILVAX; YEL/VAC.

yel/vac is an abbreviation for yellow fever vaccine.
see YELLOW FEVER VACCINE.

Yomesan (*Bayer*) is a proprietary, non-prescription form of the ANTHELMINTIC drug niclosamide, used to treat infestation by tapeworms; it is produced as chewy yellow tablets. Careful monitoring of the infestation is required, together with reassuring counselling of the patient.

▲ side-effects: see NICLOSAMIDE.

✚ warning: consumption of alcohol should be avoided during treatment.

Zadstat (*Lederle*) is a proprietary ANTIBIOTIC and
ANTIPROTOZOAL drug, available only on prescription, used
to treat infections by anaerobic bacteria or protozoa,
particularly infections of the rectum, colon and vagina. It
may also be used to treat ulcerative infections of the
gums. Produced in the form of tablets, suppositories (in
either of two strengths), and in a Minipack for
intravenous infusion, Zadstat is a preparation of the drug
metronidazole.
▲/✚ side-effects/warning: *see* METRONIDAZOLE.

Zinacef (*Glaxo*) is a proprietary broad-spectrum
ANTIBIOTIC, available only on prescription, used to treat
bacterial infections and to prevent infection arising
during and after surgery. Produced in the form of powder
for reconstitution as a medium for injections, Zinacef is a
preparation of the CEPHALOSPORIN cefuroxime.
▲/✚ side-effects/warning: *see* CEFUROXIME.

Zinamide (*Merck, Sharp & Dohme*) is a proprietary
ANTITUBERCULAR drug, available only on prescription,
consisting of tablets containing pyrazinamide. Usually
prescribed in combination with other antitubercular
drugs, it is not recommended for children.
▲/✚ side-effects/warning: *see* PYRAZINAMIDE.

Zovirax (*Wellcome*) is a proprietary form of the ANTIVIRAL
drug acyclovir, available only on prescription, used to
treat infection by herpes simplex and herpes zoster
organisms. It is available in the form of tablets (in either
of two strengths), a suspension (for dilution with syrup or
sorbitol; the potency of the diluted suspension is retained
for 28 days), and a powder for reconstitution as an
intravenous infusion. To treat one form of herpes simplex
there is also an eye ointment; urogenital forms of herpes
are treated by a water-based cream. Treatment by any of
these preparations is required at least 4 times a day.
▲/✚ side-effects/warning: *see* ACYCLOVIR.

Z